KU-541-887

Anatomy and Physiology

for holistic therapists

2nd edition

Francesca Gould

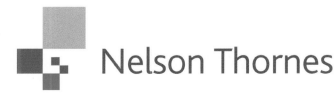
Nelson Thornes

Text © Francesca Gould 2001, 2005
Original illustrations © Nelson Thornes Ltd 2005

The right of Francesca Gould to be identified as author of this work has been asserted by her in accordance with the Copyright, Designs and Patents Act 1988.

All rights reserved. No part of this publication may be reproduced or transmitted in any form or by any means, electronic or mechanical, including photocopy, recording or any information storage and retrieval system, without permission in writing from the publisher or under licence from the Copyright Licensing Agency Limited, of Saffron House, 6–10 Kirby Street, London, EC1N 8TS.

Any person who commits any unauthorised act in relation to this publication may be liable to criminal prosecution and civil claims for damages.

The VTCT name and logo are the trade marks of VTCT and are used under licence.

First published in 2001

This edition published in 2005 by:
Nelson Thornes Ltd
Delta Place
27 Bath Road
CHELTENHAM
GL53 7TH
United Kingdom

08 09 / 10 9 8 7 6 5

A catalogue record for this book is available from the British Library

ISBN 978 0 7487 9356 3

Illustrations by Oxford Designers and Illustrators
Page make-up by Florence Production Ltd

Printed and bound in Croatia by Zrinski

ACKNOWLEDGEMENTS

The author and publishers would like to thank Janet Hesford, Heather Mole and Claire Bates for their help in the production of this book.

Contents

Foreword

I am delighted to write the foreword for *Anatomy and Physiology for Holistic Therapists*. This is yet another example of the publications which have been fully approved and endorsed by the Vocational Training Charitable Trust (VTCT) in collaboration with Nelson Thornes. VTCT is the leading awarding body in the field of Beauty and Holistic Therapy and has a growing presence in the area of Health, Fitness and Sport. As such, VTCT recognises the importance to practice in these areas of the underpinning knowledge which is provided through the study of anatomy and physiology. The VTCT Level 3 Diploma in Anatomy and Physiology is one of our most popular qualifications in Body Massage, Aromatherapy, Reflexology, Sports and Fitness Therapy and Sports Massage.

This book provides clear explanations for readers who have little or no initial background in the subject and provides sufficient knowledge for the requirements of VTCT qualifications. It is easy to read, has many illustrations and the small tasks aid the learning process. The format is very clear and the style is attractive thus making what can often be a daunting subject quite accessible. It is presented in a way which makes the information interesting and encourages the learner to persevere.

Francesca Gould has, once again, been successful in utilising her extensive experience and the broad knowledge which is required to cover this subject in order to produce a text which has great clarity, accurate information and yet provides a simple approach to the subject matter.

I hope that you find this book of great assistance to your future studies and practice, especially in Holistic Therapies but also in Sports Therapy.

Peter Wren
Chief Executive
VTCT

NOTE FROM THE AUTHOR

I have written this book primarily for VTCT and ITEC Holistic Therapist students, but it will also be a valuable tool for beauty and sports therapy students. It is essential to have a good knowledge of anatomy and physiology to be a successful therapist. As a lecturer and practising therapist, I wanted to impart my knowledge to produce a book which was written clearly and simply. To facilitate learning I have included tasks such as crosswords to make the subject fun. Anatomy and Physiology, although extremely interesting is a vast subject with many long words to learn! I hope this book will help to alleviate fear and make the subject an enjoyable one.

Francesca Gould

Cells

Fact!

The body is made up of
100,000 billion cells.

To help you understand the systems of the body, it is necessary first of all to have knowledge of the cell. Like the bricks of a house, cells are the building blocks of the body.

The body is made up of 100,000 billion cells. Although minute, cells are organised and complex structures. Different cells have certain functions, such as muscle, blood and fat cells, and can vary in size and shape. Groups of **cells** together make **tissues** and a group of tissues become an **organ**. A **system** is made up of various organs, such as the cardiovascular system.

- **Cell**, e.g. a heart muscle cell (Figure 1.1)
- **Tissue**, e.g. heart muscle tissue (Figure 1.2)
- **Organ**, e.g. the heart (Figure 1.3)
- **System**, e.g. the circulatory system (Figure 1.4)

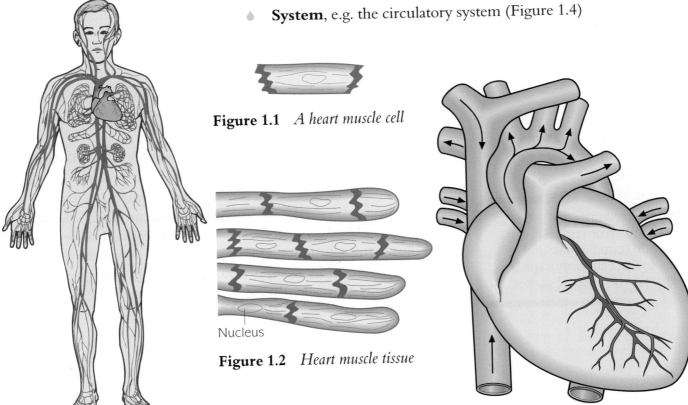

Figure 1.1 *A heart muscle cell*

Nucleus

Figure 1.2 *Heart muscle tissue*

Figure 1.3 *The heart*

Figure 1.4 *The circulatory system*

Structure of cells

Nearly all cells have the same basic structure. They are surrounded by a ① **membrane**, which encloses the contents of the cell. Cells contain organelles (small organs), which are responsible for the functioning of a cell.

② **Cytoplasm** is a jelly-like liquid consisting mostly of water, but it also contains nutrients required by the cell for growth, reproduction and repair. The cytoplasm contains many organelles.

The ③ **nucleus** is the largest organelle and is surrounded by the nuclear membrane. The function of the nucleus is to control the cell's activities. The processes that occur in each cell can be likened to workers in a factory. Therefore, the nucleus is the managing director of a cell.

Almost all cells have a nucleus, which contains chromosomes. Chromosomes are strings of DNA (deoxyribonucleic acid) and carry all the information needed to make an entire human being. Within the nucleus will be the ④ **nucleolus**. It is a dense area of almost pure DNA.

There are two types of **endoplasmic reticulum** (ER): smooth and rough:

- ⑤ **Smooth ER** produces and transports fats, known as steroids and lipids. The hormones oestrogen and testosterone are produced by the smooth ER.

- ⑥ **Rough ER** is covered with tiny granules called **ribosomes**. The function of ribosomes is to make protein. The rough ER transports these proteins through the cytoplasm to the ⑦ **Golgi body**, also known as Golgi apparatus. The Golgi body sorts and packages the proteins. Some proteins will be used inside the cell and other proteins, such as hormones and enzymes, will be transported out of the cell. Many structures in the body are made from protein, such as keratin found in hair and nails.

Lysosomes are the cell's waste disposal units. They are little sacs that release substances called enzymes to destroy bacteria, worn out parts of the cell and other unwanted substances.

Sausage-shaped organelles called ⑧ **mitochondria** (singular: mitochondrion) are the powerhouses and help to produce energy

Fact!

Chromosomes are strings of DNA (deoxyribonucleic acid) and carry all the information needed to make an entire human being.

Note

Many structures in the body are made from protein, e.g. keratin found in hair and nails. The cell membrane is also partly made of protein.

Cells that require little energy to carry out their functions, e.g. fat cells, have few mitochondria. The cells that use a lot of energy, e.g. muscle and liver cells, have many mitochondria.

for the cell. Cells that require little energy to carry out their functions, e.g. fat cells, have few mitochondria. The cells that use a lot of energy, e.g. muscle and liver cells, have many mitochondria.

⑨ **Vacuoles** are empty spaces which store and transport substances such as waste products and water.

Task 1.1

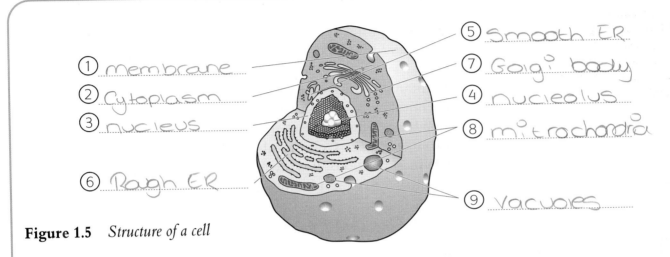

① membrane
② Cytoplasm
③ nucleus
⑥ Rogh ER

⑤ Smooth ER
⑦ Golgi body
④ nucieolus
⑧ mitrochondria
⑨ Vacuoles

Figure 1.5 *Structure of a cell*

Label the diagram in Figure 1.5 matching the numbers to the numbered terms in the text above and on page 2. Use this key to colour the diagram:

Blue – cell membrane
Yellow – cytoplasm
Red – nucleus

Green – Golgi body
Orange – mitochondria
Brown – ER.

Cellular respiration

For the cells to produce energy to carry out their work they require fuel. The food we eat provides the fuel. It is absorbed from the intestines into the bloodstream. Tiny food molecules, e.g. glucose, eventually pass into the tissue fluid – this is fluid that surrounds and nourishes the cells. The process whereby fuel molecules are broken down and energy is released is known as **cellular respiration**.

Glucose is a type of sugar which is produced when the body breaks down carbohydrates from foods such as potatoes and bread.

Glucose is the fuel mostly used by the cell, although other foods such as fat and protein can be used if there is a glucose shortage.

Oxygen is also vital for cells to burn up the glucose. Oxygen enters the body through the lungs and passes into the bloodstream. The oxygen passes into the tissue fluid that surrounds the cells. Cells use the glucose and oxygen to make energy for the cell's activities.

When cells respire they form the by-products carbon dioxide and water. Carbon dioxide is a gas that is toxic to the body, so it is removed by the blood and taken to the lungs to be breathed out. The water is utilised by the body.

Without glucose and oxygen the cells would die, as the many chemical reactions constantly taking place inside the cell would stop happening. These chemical reactions are important for maintaining life. **Cell metabolism** is the sum total of all these chemical reactions. It is the production of energy in the cell that is essential for cell respiration, growth and division.

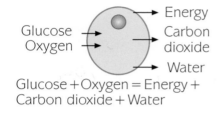

Glucose + Oxygen = Energy + Carbon dioxide + Water

Figure 1.6 *Cellular respiration*

Basal metabolic rate

Energy is required for activities of the body such as breathing, digestion, heartbeat and the functioning of the brain. The **basal metabolic rate (BMR)** is the minimum energy needed to keep the body alive. Food and drink provide the energy in the form of calories. The daily intake of energy should equal the energy needs of metabolism; otherwise a person will gain or lose weight. The amount required can be measured in people at complete rest.

Daily requirements for a man are:

- at rest – around 2,000 calories
- for sedentary work – around 2,500 calories
- for heavy manual work – around 3,500 calories.

Cell membrane

The cell membrane consists of mainly lipids (fat) and some protein. It is partially permeable, i.e. it will only allow certain substances to pass through it. The membrane controls and regulates what gets into and out of the cell.

Fact!

- Generally, the heavier the body, the higher the basal metabolic rate as more energy will be needed to maintain it and move it about.

- Men generally need more calories each day than women.

Note

Molecules are made up of atoms joined together. For example: CO_2 (carbon dioxide) has one carbon atom (C) and two oxygen atoms (O_2). The joining of the carbon atom and the oxygen atoms makes one molecule.

Diffusion

The process by which small molecules such as oxygen and carbon dioxide pass through the cell membrane is known as **diffusion**. Diffusion is the movement of molecules from an area of high concentration (where there are lots of them) to an area of low concentration (where there are fewer).

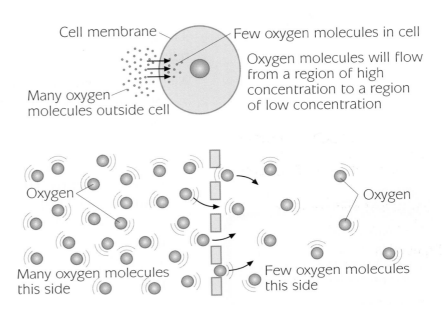

Figure 1.7 *Diffusion*

Osmosis

Osmosis involves the movement of water molecules from a region of higher concentration of water to a region of lower concentration of water through a partially permeable membrane, such as the cell membrane.

If the cell contains little water compared to the surrounding tissue fluid, it will draw water into the cell from the tissue fluid by **osmosis**. If the cell contains too much water compared to the tissue fluid, then excess will pass into the tissue fluid.

Figure 1.8 *Osmosis*

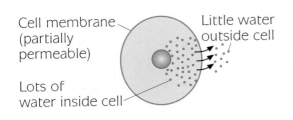

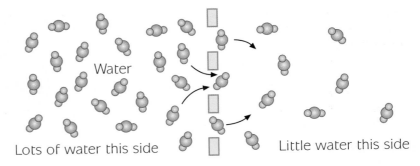

Cell division (mitosis)

A cell does not keep on growing in size but divides into two daughter cells. The cells further multiply by splitting in half again and again. The cells continue to divide until the billions of cells needed to make up the body are produced. This process of cell division is called **mitosis**. Mitosis of cells is also needed for growth and the replacement of dead cells.

The growth and division of a cell consists of five phases (the letters refer to Figure 1.9):

A   The cell spends most of its life in **interphase**. During this phase the cell actively grows.

B   **Prophase** is the first phase of mitosis, the **chromatin** (strands of genetic material) coil tightly to form dark X-shaped structures, known as **chromosomes**. They are arranged in pairs, called **chromatids**, and are attached to the **centromere**. During prophase, the nucleus becomes smaller and disappears. Two pairs of organelles called **centrioles** go toward each end of the cell and form cell fibres, also known as spindles.

C   During **metaphase**, chromosomes line up in the middle of the cell.

> **Note**
>
> The centrosome is an area found in the centre of a cell in which tube-like structures called centrioles are found.

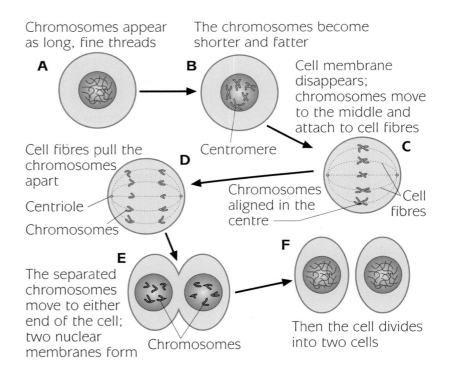

Figure 1.9 *Mitosis*

D During **anaphase**, the chromatids separate and become individual chromosomes, rather than a pair. One set of chromosomes moves to one end of the cell and the other set to the opposite end. So there are 46 chromosomes on each side.

E,F **Telophase** now begins. A nuclear membrane starts to form around each set of chromosomes. The cell will begin to constrict around its middle and then divide to form two cells.

Meiosis

To make a human being, 46 chromosomes are needed. There are only 23 chromosomes in an egg and 23 chromosomes in a sperm (as these sex cells undergo a special process called **meiosis**, their number of chromosomes is halved). When fertilisation takes place, the egg and sperm join together (so result in 46 chromosomes) and form a **zygote**. The zygote is able to reproduce by cell division (mitosis).

> **Note**
>
> The microscopic study of tissues is called **histology**.

Homeostasis

For each cell to carry out its functions, the body must maintain a constant internal environment, known as **homeostasis**. Homeostasis is the basis of good health. The healthy body shows regular biological rhythms, such as sleeping and waking patterns and monthly periods in women.

The hypothalamus in the brain is one of the main regulators of homeostasis. It controls body temperature, hunger, thirst and emotional behaviour, such as rage, pleasure, fear and sexual behaviour.

The main organs concerned with homeostasis are the lungs, skin, liver and kidneys. There are different bodily activities that need to be controlled, which include the sugar levels, water levels, salt levels and temperature. These are all important to the body but need to be at just the right levels, not too high or low otherwise problems can occur.

pH balance in the body

A pH reading indicates if a fluid is acid or alkaline. Body fluids have pH values that should remain relatively constant for normal cell activity to occur.

The division of cells leads to a big group of cells being formed, which is known as **tissue**. Different types of tissue have specific functions in the body.

Epithelial tissue

This kind of tissue provides protective covering for surfaces inside and outside the body. There are two types of epithelial tissue, simple and compound.

Simple epithelial tissue

This type of tissue consists of a single layer of cells and includes:

- **Pavement** or **squamous epithelial cells**, which are flat, thin cells placed edge to edge, like the slabs of a pavement. Their thinness allows for rapid movement of substances through them. These cells are found in the alveoli (air sacs) of the lungs, in the lining of the heart and in blood and lymph vessels.

- **Columnar cells**, which are tall, column-shaped cells. They line the ducts of most glands, the gall bladder and nearly the whole of the digestive tract.

- **Cuboidal cells**, which consist of cube-shaped cells and can be found covering the ovaries, in the kidneys and within the eye. They are involved in absorbing and releasing substances.

- **Ciliated cells**, which are columnar in shape but have the addition of fine, hair-like structures called cilia attached at the head. These cells line the respiratory passages and also the oviducts (Fallopian tubes). In the respiratory tract, the constant movement of the cilia help to prevent dust and bacteria from entering the lungs. In the Fallopian tubes, cilia help move the ovum (egg) along the tube.

Compound epithelial tissue

This type of tissue consists of two or more layers. There are two types of compound tissue:

- **Stratified epithelium** (stratified = in layers), which consists of two or more layers of cells. It is more durable and can protect underlying tissues from the external environment and wear and tear. It forms the top five layers of the skin known as the epidermal layers. It also lines the mouth, throat, food pipe, the anal canal and the vagina and covers the surface of the eye.

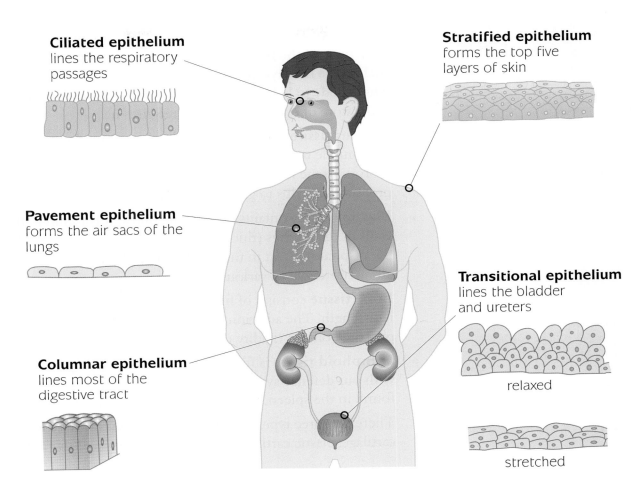

Simple

Ciliated epithelium
lines the respiratory
passages

Pavement epithelium
forms the air sacs of the
lungs

Columnar epithelium
lines most of the
digestive tract

Compound

Stratified epithelium
forms the top five
layers of skin

Transitional epithelium
lines the bladder
and ureters

relaxed

stretched

Figure 1.10 *Epithelial tissue*

● **Transitional epithelium**, which is variable in appearance, depending on whether it is relaxed or stretched, and consists of several layers of cells. It lines the bladder and ureters (tubes entering the bladder from the kidneys). Its function is to help prevent rupture of organs.

Connective tissue

The function of connective tissue is to protect, bind and support. There are several types:

● **Areolar tissue** is widely distributed throughout the body. It consists of a watery gel supporting a network of fine, white fibres. These fibres are made of collagen which gives the tissue strength. It forms a thin, transparent tissue surrounding vessels (such as a blood vessel that carries blood), nerves and muscle fibres in muscle. It also has the function of connecting skin to

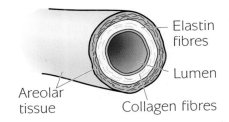

Elastin
fibres

Lumen

Areolar
tissue

Collagen fibres

Figure 1.11 *Areolar tissue*

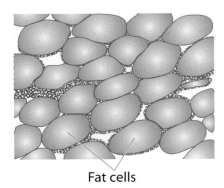

Fat cells

Figure 1.12 *Adipose tissue*

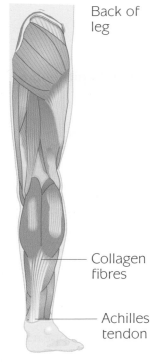

Back of leg

Collagen fibres

Achilles tendon

Figure 1.13 *Fibrous tissue*

tissues and muscles. Areolar tissue also contains stretchy fibres of elastin protein.

🔹 **Adipose tissue** consists of fat cells. This fatty tissue is found in most parts of the body. It helps to support and protect organs, such as the kidneys. It forms a protective covering for the whole body to help protect against injury, provides insulation and a store of energy if the body requires it.

🔹 **Fibrous tissue** is found in muscles, bones, tendons (which join muscle to bone) and ligaments (which join bone to bone). Fibrous tissue is made of collagen fibres; collagen is a type of protein that helps to give strength to the tissues.

🔹 **Elastic tissue** contains elastic-type fibres. It is found in the walls of the arteries (thick blood vessels) and in the air tubes of the respiratory tract in the chest, where elasticity is needed to allow stretching of various organs.

🔹 **Bone tissue** consists of fibrous material, which gives the bone its strength. The addition of salts, such as calcium phosphate, give the bone its rigidity (see Chapter 3).

🔹 **Lymphoid tissue** is found in lymph nodes (lymph nodes help with our defence system and inflame when infected). It is also found in the spleen, tonsils and appendix.(See Chapter 5.)

🔹 There are three types of **cartilage** found in the body: hyaline cartilage, elastic cartilage and fibrocartilage (see Table 1.1).

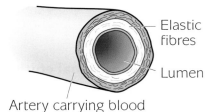

Elastic fibres

Lumen

Artery carrying blood

Figure 1.14 *Elastic tissue*

Table 1.1 *Types of cartilage*

Cartilage	Description	Where found in body
Hyaline cartilage	Most common type of cartilage found in body. It is firm, elastic and reduces friction and absorbs shock at joints.	At joints. The C-shaped rings that keep the windpipe open.
Elastic cartilage	Also called yellow elastic cartilage as it contains yellow elastic fibres. It is flexible and readily springs back into shape.	At the tip of the nose and the upper part of the ear (the earlobe is made of adipose and fibrous tissue).
Fibrocartilage	Also known as white fibrocartilage and made up of bundles of fibres with cartilage cells inbetween.	Where great strength is required, such as in the discs between the bones that form the spine.

Membranes

There are three types of membrane in the body: mucous, synovial and serous (see Table 1.2).

Table 1.2 *Types of membrane*

Membrane	Description	Where found in body
Mucous membrane	Produces a slimy, sticky fluid called mucus, which lubricates the surfaces and prevents them from drying out.	Lines the surfaces in the body that open to the outside, such as the digestive tract, air passages, urinary tract and reproductive tract.
Synovial membrane	Produces a thick fluid, rather like egg white, called synovial fluid. The fluid cushions and lubricates the ends of the bones.	Lines the spaces around certain joints, such as the knee joint.
Serous membrane	Produces a watery fluid called serous fluid, which enables organs to slide freely against each other to prevent friction.	Surrounds the lungs, the heart and the organs in the abdomen.

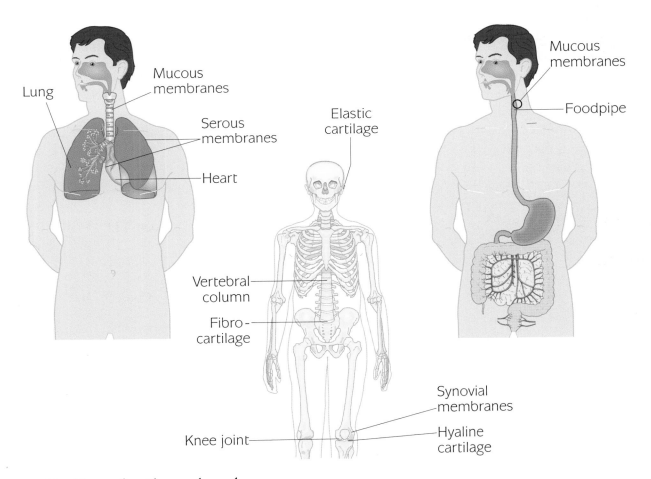

Figure 1.15 *Types of cartilage and membrane*

Match the terms in the bubbles with the correct description in the list:

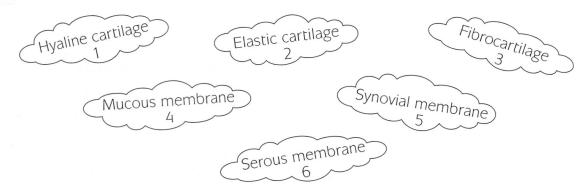

- Produces fluid to enable organs to slide freely over each other ....
- Produces mucus, which prevents surfaces from drying out ....
- Helps to absorb shock at joints ....
- Produces a thick fluid and is found at joints ....
- Found where great strength is needed, such as between the discs in the backbone ....
- Flexible and springy and found in the upper part of the ear ....

The skin

2

The skin is a large organ and forms a protective, waterproof covering over the entire surface of the body. It is thinnest on the eyelids and thickest on the soles of the feet. The skin is continually shedding and renewing itself. It is made up of layers called the **epidermis**, **dermis** and **subcutaneous layer**.

EPIDERMIS

The upper portion of the skin consists of five layers and is known as the epidermis.

Task 2.1

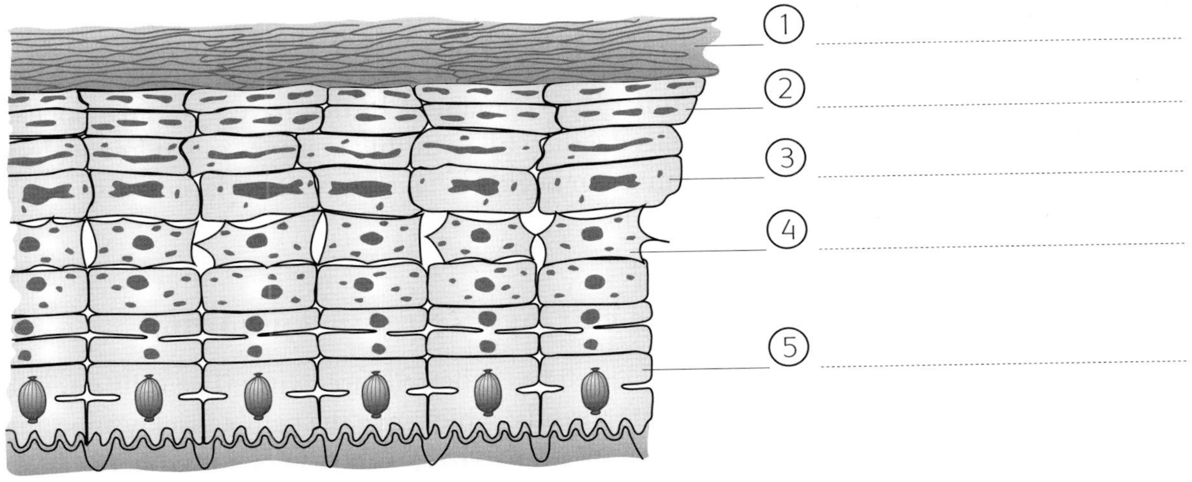

Figure 2.1 *The epidermis*

Label the diagram in Figure 2.1 matching the numbers to the numbered terms in the following text. Use this key to colour the diagram:

Yellow – layers 1 and 2

Red and yellow (i.e. some cells red, some yellow) – layer 3

Red – layers 4 and 5.

Fact!

About 80 per cent of house dust consists of dead skin cells.

① Horny layer (stratum corneum)

The top layer of the epidermis is called the horny layer, and consists of flat, overlapping, **keratinised** cells. Keratin is a protein responsible for the hardening process (keratinisation) that cells undergo when they change from living cells with a nucleus to dead cells without a nucleus. Cells that have undergone keratinisation are therefore dead.

The keratinised cells help to prevent bacteria entering through the skin and protect the body from minor injury. Cells of the horny layer are continually being rubbed off the body by friction and are replaced by cells from the layers beneath. The shedding of dead skin cells is known as **desquamation**.

② Clear layer (stratum lucidum)

The clear layer is found below the horny layer and consists of dead, keratinised cells without a nucleus. The cells are transparent, which allows the passage of sunlight into the deeper layers. This layer is only found on the fingertips, the palms of the hands and the soles of the feet.

③ Granular layer (stratum granulosum)

The granular layer contains cells that have a granular appearance. As the cells die they fill with tiny granules called **keratohyalin** and so keratinisation begins to take place. This layer consists of living and dead cells.

Note

To help you remember the layers of the epidermis, depending on which names you need to learn, think of:

Happy – horny
Clever – clear
Girls – granular
Pat – prickle cell
Back – basal

or

Corny – stratum **corn**eum
Lucy's – stratum **luci**dum
Granny – stratum **gran**ulosum
Spins – stratum **spin**osum
Germs – stratum **germ**inativum.

④ Prickle cell layer (stratum spinosum)

In the prickle cell layer the cells are living. The cells interlock by arm-like fine threads, which give the cells a prickly appearance. Pigment granules called **melanin** may be found here.

⑤ Basal layer (stratum germinativum)

The basal layer is the deepest layer in the epidermis and is in contact with the dermis directly beneath it. These cells are living, contain a nucleus and divide (mitosis) to make new skin cells. As new cells are produced they push older cells above them towards the surface of the skin, until they finally reach the horny layer. It takes 3–6 weeks for the skin cells to be pushed up from the basal layer to the horny layer.

Skin pigmentation

Cells called **melanocytes** are found within the basal layer and produce granules of melanin. Melanin is responsible for the pigment (colour) of the skin and is stimulated by ultraviolet rays from the sun. This is why the skin develops a tan after sunbathing. Its function is to protect the deeper layers of the skin from damage. Approximately 1 in every 10 basal cells is a melanocyte. Everyone has the same amount of melanocytes but produces varying quantities of melanin. This will determine the depth of skin colour. More melanin is produced in black skins than white skins, and this extra protection can help black skins to age more slowly than white skins.

DERMIS

Below the epidermis lies the dermis, which connects with the basal layer. It consists of two layers:

⬧ The upper section is called the **papillary layer** and contains small tubes called **capillaries**, which carry blood and lymph;

Task 2.2

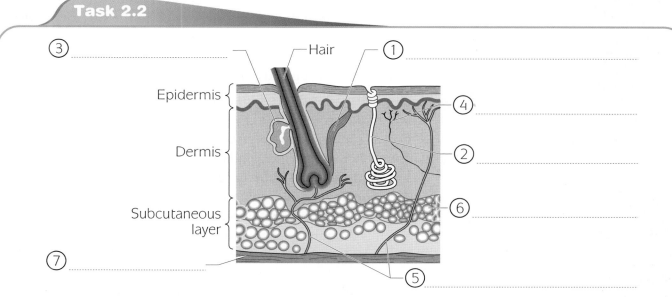

Figure 2.2 *The skin and its structures*

Label the diagram in Figure 2.2 matching the numbers to the numbered terms in the following text. Use this key to colour the diagram:

Pink – arrector pili muscle and the muscle below the subcutaneous layer
Blue – sweat gland
Yellow – adipose tissue and sebaceous gland.
Red – blood vessels.

there are also nerve endings. This layer provides nutrients for the living layers of the epidermis.

◆ The **reticular layer** contains many connective tissue fibres. Collagen gives the skin strength and elastin gives the skin its elasticity. Wavy bands of tough collagen fibres restrict the extent to which the skin can be stretched, and elastic fibres return the skin back to shape after it has been stretched.

The dermis also contains nerves, hair follicles, sebaceous glands, sweat glands and arrector pili; these are known as **appendages**.

① **Arrector pili** muscles are small muscles attached to the hair follicles. When we are cold the contraction of these muscles causes the hairs to stand on end. This results in the appearance of goose bumps. Air is trapped between the skin and hair and is warmed by body heat. This can help to keep the body warm.

There are two types of sweat gland in the body:

◆ ② **Eccrine glands** excrete sweat and are found all over the body. The sweat duct opens directly on to the surface of the skin through an opening called a **pore**. Sweat is a mixture of water, salt and toxins. Black skins contain larger and more numerous sweat glands than white skins.

◆ **Apocrine glands** are found in the armpits, around the nipples and in the groin area. They secrete a milky substance. These glands are larger than eccrine glands and are attached to the hair follicle. Apocrine glands are controlled by hormones, becoming active at puberty. Body odour is caused by the breaking down of the apocrine sweat by bacteria. Substances called pheromones are present in this milky substance; the smell is thought to play a part in sexual attraction between individuals and the recognition of mothers by their babies.

③ **Sebaceous glands** are small, sac-like structures which produce a substance called **sebum**. Sebum is a fatty substance and is the skin's natural moisturiser. These glands are found all over the body, but are more numerous on the scalp and areas of the face such as the nose, forehead and chin. Hormones control the activity of these glands and as we get older the secretion of sebum decreases, causing the skin to become drier. Sebum and sweat mix together on the skin to form an **acid mantle**. The acid mantle maintains the pH (acid/alkaline level) of the skin at 5.5–5.6; this helps to protect the skin from harmful bacteria. Some soaps can affect the acid mantle and cause irritation and drying of the skin.

Note

To help you remember the position of the sweat glands think of **E** (eccrine glands) for **everywhere** and **A** (apocrine glands) for **armpits**.

Note

A third of all toxins are expelled from the body through sweat, therefore the skin helps to detoxify the body. A build-up of toxins may be the cause of many skin conditions.

Note

Apocrine glands are also found on the feet.

④ **Sensory nerve endings** are found all over the body but are particularly numerous on our fingertips and lips. These nerves will make us aware of feelings of pain, touch, heat and cold by sending messages through sensory nerves to the brain.

Messages are sent from the brain through **motor nerves**. Motor nerves stimulate the sweat glands, arrector pili muscles and sebaceous glands to carry out their functions.

Blood within the ⑤ **blood vessels** provides the skin with oxygen and nutrients. The living cells of the skin produce waste products such as carbon dioxide and metabolic waste. These waste products pass from the cells and enter into the bloodstream to be taken away and removed by the body.

SUBCUTANEOUS LAYER

The subcutaneous layer is situated below the dermis. It consists of ⑥ **adipose tissue** (fat) and areolar tissue. The adipose tissue helps to protect the body against injury and acts as an insulating layer against heat loss, helping to keep the body warm. The areolar tissue contains elastic fibres, making this layer elastic and flexible.
⑦ **Muscle** is situated below the subcutaneous layer and is attached to bone.

FUNCTIONS OF THE SKIN

Sensation

The skin contains sensory nerve endings that send messages to the brain. These nerves respond to touch, pressure, pain, cold and heat and allow us to recognise objects from their feel and shape.

Heat regulation

It is important for the body to have a constant internal temperature of 36.8 degrees Celsius (°C). The skin helps to maintain this temperature by:

- **Vasoconstriction** This occurs when the body becomes cold. The blood vessels constrict reducing the flow of blood through the capillaries. Heat lost from the surface of the skin is therefore reduced.

- **Vasodilation** This occurs when the body becomes too hot. The capillaries expand and the blood flow increases; this allows heat to be lost from the body by radiation.

Match up the bubbles with the correct definition in the list:

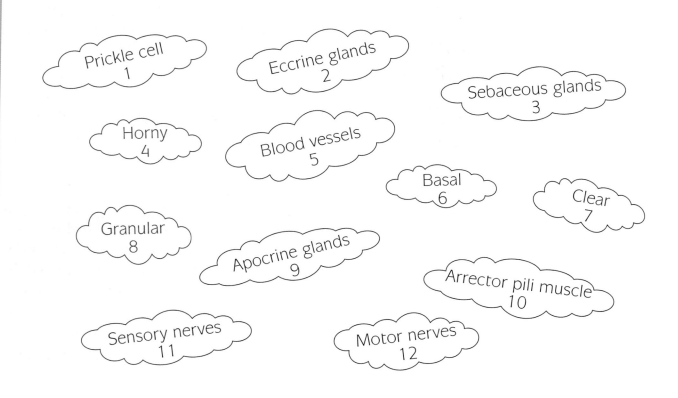

Prickle cell
1

Eccrine glands
2

Sebaceous glands
3

Horny
4

Blood vessels
5

Basal
6

Clear
7

Granular
8

Apocrine glands
9

Arrector pili muscle
10

Sensory nerves
11

Motor nerves
12

- Process of keratinisation takes place here ....
- Dead cells of this layer are rubbed off by friction ....
- Contracts causing hair to stand on end ....
- Layer found on palms of hands and soles of feet ....
- Send messages informing the brain about the sensations of pain, hot and cold
  ....
- Deepest layer in epidermis and in contact with the dermis ....
- Found all over the body and excrete sweat ....
- Stimulate sweat glands and sebaceous glands to carry out their
  functions ....
- Releases a moisturising substance called sebum ....
- Living cell with a prickly appearance ....
- Release milky substance and found in armpits and groin area ....
- Bring supplies of oxygen and nutrients vital to skin ....

- **Goose bumps** Contraction of the arrector pili muscle when we are cold causes the hairs to stand on end, keeping a layer of warm air close to the body. This was probably of more use to our ancestors, who were generally hairier.

- **Shivering** Shivering when we are cold helps to warm the body, as the contraction of the muscles produces heat within the body.

- **Sweating** In hot conditions the rate of sweat production increases. The eccrine glands excrete sweat onto the skin surface and heat is lost as the water evaporates from the skin.

Absorption

The skin is largely waterproof and absorbs very little, although certain substances are able to pass through the basal layer. Essential oils can pass through the hair follicles and into the bloodstream. Certain medications such as hormone replacement therapy can be given through patches placed on the skin. Ultraviolet rays from the sun are also able to penetrate through the basal layer.

Protection

The skin protects the body by keeping harmful bacteria out and provides a covering for all the organs inside. It also protects underlying structures from the harmful effects of ultraviolet (UV) light. The other functions of the skin also help to protect the body.

Excretion

Eccrine glands excrete sweat on to the skin's surface. Sweat consists of 99.4 per cent water, 0.4 per cent toxins and 0.2 per cent salts.

Secretion

Sebum is a fatty substance secreted from the sebaceous gland on to the skin's surface. It keeps the skin supple and helps to waterproof it.

Vitamin D

The UV rays from the sun penetrate through the skin's layers and activate a chemical found in the skin called ergosterol, which changes into vitamin D. Vitamin D is essential for healthy bones and deficiency can cause rickets, a condition in which the bones are malformed.

> **Note**
>
> A good way of remembering the functions of the skin is the words **SHAPES VD**:
>
> **S** – **s**ensation
> **H** – **h**eat regulation
> **A** – **a**bsorption
> **P** – **p**rotection
> **E** – **e**xcretion
> **S** – **s**ecretion
> **VD** – **v**itamin D formation.

Fill in the gaps in the following text.

- .... nerve endings respond to touch, pressure and pain. They send the information to the brain.
- It is important for the body temperature to remain at ....
- To reduce heat loss from the skin the blood vessels .... This is known as vasoconstriction.
- When the body becomes too hot the capillaries dilate so heat can be lost. This is known as ....
- Goose bumps are caused by the contraction of the .... muscles.
- Shivering helps to .... the body because of the contraction of the muscles.
- Sweating helps to .... the body as heat is lost as the sweat evaporates.
- The skin can absorb certain substances, including the following: ...., ... and ....
- Sweat consists of water, ... and ....
- A fatty substance called .... is secreted on to the skin's surface.
- Vitamin ....production is stimulated by the penetration of UV rays through the skin.

EFFECTS OF MASSAGE ON THE SKIN

- The circulation is improved and so fresh blood brings nutrients to the sebaceous glands; therefore sebum production is increased. Sebum helps to make the skin soft and supple.

- The sweat glands become more active and so more sweat is excreted. Toxins such as urea and other waste products are eliminated from the body in this way.

- Massage also causes the top layer of dead skin cells to be shed (desquamation), which improves the condition of the skin, giving it a healthy glow.

- The sensory nerve endings can either be soothed or stimulated, depending on the massage movements used.

- When massage and essential oils are used together, the skin's health and appearance can be greatly improved.

SKIN AGEING

When a person is in their early twenties, the skin should be at its best. In the late twenties and early thirties, fine lines appear on the skin's surface, especially around the eyes where the skin is thinner.

After 40 years, hormone activity in the body slows down so the sebaceous glands produce less sebum and the skin becomes increasingly drier. Lines and wrinkles appear on the surface. Wrinkling is due to changes in the collagen and elastin fibres of the connective tissue. The collagen fibres in the dermis begin to decrease in number, stiffen and break apart. The elastin fibres lose some of their elasticity and break down, so that when the skin is stretched it does not immediately return to its original state when stretching stops. In people who are regularly exposed to ultraviolet light or who smoke, the loss of elasticity of the skin is greatly accelerated. Constant facial expressions cause crow's feet to be found at the sides of the eyes.

In the late fifties, brown patches of discoloured skin called lentigines (liver spots) may appear because of an increase in the size of some melanocytes. Liver spots are commonly seen around the temple areas of the face and on the backs of the hands. The blood flow to the skin is reduced and the rate of mitosis in the basal layer slows down. The horny layer is therefore thinner, making the skin more fragile. Dilated capillaries appear, especially on the cheeks and nose.

Sebaceous glands decrease in size, which leads to dry and cracked skin. The sweat glands are less active and loss of subcutaneous fat often occurs. The hair growth slows down and a decrease in the number of functioning melanocytes results in grey hairs. The skin of older people heals poorly and becomes more susceptible to infection and also skin cancer.

Task 2.5

List five changes that take place in the skin as it ages.

1 ....

2 ....

3 ....

4 ....

5 ....

Factors affecting the condition of the skin

Ageing of the skin may occur naturally or it may prematurely age because of various factors, including heredity, environment (perhaps work outside in all weathers), inadequate diet, smoking or ill-health.

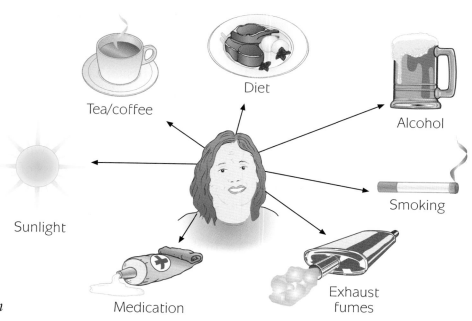

Figure 2.3 *Factors affecting the skin*

Diet

The best nutritional recommendation to ensure healthy skin is to eat a well-balanced diet. The Western diet generally contains the essential vitamins and minerals required for a healthy skin. These include vitamins A, B_3 (niacin) and C. Vitamin A helps to control the rate of keratinisation in the skin and so deficiency of this vitamin can result in dry skin. If the diet is deficient in vitamin B_3 a disease called pellagra can occur; one of its features is dermatitis. Vitamin C is required by the body to produce collagen and deficiency of this vitamin can also lead to dermatitis.

Alcohol is not harmful to the skin in moderation but large amounts dilate the blood vessels and over time may weaken the capillary walls and lead to broken capillaries and redness; this can often be seen on the face. Alcohol also dehydrates the skin by drawing water from the tissues and robbing the body of vitamins B and C, which are required for a healthy skin.

Caffeine is found in tea, coffee and some fizzy soft drinks. In moderate doses it will cause no harm but excessive amounts can interfere with the absorption of vitamins and minerals, which can result in an unhealthy skin.

Sunlight

Ultraviolet radiation from the sun penetrates the dermis of the skin and causes damage. It causes dehydration and also interferes with the structure of the collagen and elastin fibres. The skin loses its strength and elasticity, resulting in severe wrinkling and sagging, especially noticeable in people who spend a great deal of time in the sun.

Smoking

Smoking interferes with cell respiration and slows down the blood circulation as nicotine is a vasoconstrictor. This makes it harder for nutrients to reach the skin cells and for waste products to be eliminated. Cigarette smoking also releases a chemical that destroys vitamin C. This interferes with the production of collagen and so contributes to premature ageing. People who have smoked for a long time will generally look 10 years older than non-smokers of the same age.

Medication

Certain medications taken by mouth can lead to skin dehydration, fluid retention or swelling of the tissues – steroids are an example. Hydrocortisone creams are applied externally and are used to treat skin conditions such as psoriasis and dermatitis. The cream should be used for short lengths of time and in small quantities otherwise thinning of the skin may result.

Antibiotics can cause temporary drying of the skin, although it will improve after the course of drugs has finished.

Taking the contraceptive pill can cause a condition known as **chloasma**, in which areas of increased pigmentation occur on the skin, usually on the face.

Environment

The moisture content of the epidermis can be affected by factors such as central heating, which creates a dry environment. This causes moisture to be lost from the epidermis and can lead to dehydration.

Air pollution from industry, car fumes, etc. harms the skin and causes dehydration.

If a person alternates between a cold and a warm environment, the capillaries contract and dilate to adapt to that particular temperature. The capillary walls become weak and this leads to permanently dilated capillaries, also called thread veins. These can commonly be seen on the cheeks and nose. There are also many other causes of dilated capillaries.

Task 2.6

Fill in the gaps in the following text.

- Vitamin ...... is required by the body to produce collagen.
- Excessive alcohol intake can lead to weakening of the .... walls.
- UV rays cause .... of the skin and also damage the structure of the .... and .... fibres.
- Smoking causes a chemical to be released that destroys vitamin ....
- Long-term smokers are more prone to .... ageing than non-smokers.
- Long-term use of hydrocortisone creams can cause ....of the skin.
- While using antibiotics the skin can become ....
- Central heating and air pollution can lead to the skin becoming ....
- If the skin alternates between cold and warm environments, damage to the capillaries may result which leads to permanently dilated capillaries called ....

SKIN TYPES

Skin types vary from person to person and can be described as being normal, dry, oily, combination, sensitive, dehydrated or mature. Essential oils can be chosen to suit each individual skin type.

Normal

This skin type will look healthy, clear and fresh. It is often seen in children, as external factors and ageing have not yet affected the condition of the skin, although the increased activity of hormones at puberty may cause the skin to become greasy.

A normal skin type will look neither oily nor dry and will have a fine, even texture. The pores are small and the skin's elasticity is good so it feels soft and firm to the touch. It is usually free of spots and blemishes.

Dry

This skin type is thin and fine and dilated capillaries can often be seen around the cheek and nose areas. The skin will feel and look dry because little sebum is being produced and it is also lacking in moisture. This skin type will often tighten after washing and there may be some dry, flaky patches. There will be no spots or comedones (blackheads) and no visible open pores. This skin type is prone to premature wrinkling, especially around the eyes, mouth and neck.

Oily

This skin type will look shiny, dull and slightly yellowish (sallow) in colour because of the excess sebum production. Oily skin is coarse, thick and will feel greasy. Enlarged pores can be seen; these are due to the excess production and build-up of sebum. Open pores can let in bacteria, which cause spots and infections. Blocked pores often lead to comedones (blackheads). Oily skin tends to age more slowly as the grease absorbs some of the UV rays and so can protect against its damaging effects. The sebum also helps to keep the skin moisturised and prevents drying.

Combination

With this skin type there will be areas of dry, normal and greasy skin. Usually the forehead, nose and chin are greasy and are known as the T-zone. The areas around the eyes and cheeks are usually dry and may be sensitive.

Sensitive

This skin type is often dry, transparent and reddens easily when touched. Dilated capillaries may be present, especially on the cheeks, which gives the face a high, red colour known as couperose skin. Hereditary factors may be a cause of sensitive skin. A skin that is sensitive may be easily irritated by certain substances so care should be taken when choosing products for this type. If a white skin is sensitive to a product it will show as a reddened area, but on black skin it will show up as a darkened area.

Dehydrated

This skin type lacks moisture and so is dry. The causes include illness, medication, too much sun, dieting and working in a dry environment with low humidity, such as an air-conditioned office.

Sebum helps to prevent evaporation of water from the skin, so when insufficient sebum is produced, moisture is lost from the skin. The skin feels and looks dry and tight. There may be flaking and fine lines present on the skin. Dilated capillaries are also common with this skin type.

Mature

This skin type is dry as the sebaceous and sweat glands become less active. The skin may be thin and wrinkles will be present. There are usually dilated capillaries, often around the nose and cheek areas. The bone structure can become more prominent as the adipose and supportive tissue become thinner. Muscle tone is often poor so the contours of the face become slack. Because of the poor blood circulation, waste products are removed less quickly so the skin may become puffy and pale in colour. Liver spots may also appear on the face and hands. The cause of this skin type is ageing and altered hormone activity.

Task 2.7

Write the characteristics of each skin type into the table below.

Skin type	Brief description
Normal	
Dry	
Oily	
Combination	
Sensitive	
Dehydrated	
Mature	

Skin diseases and disorders can be classified as bacterial infections, viral infections, fungal infections, infestations, allergies and non-infectious conditions. Some infections, such as ringworm and athlete's foot, can be caught by direct contact with an infected person. Infections can also be caught by indirect contact with contaminated items such as towels, coins, door handles, crockery etc., which can store germs such as bacteria.

Bacterial infections

Bacteria are single-celled organisms and can multiply very quickly. They are capable of breeding outside the body so can be caught easily by direct contact or by touching a contaminated article.

There are two types of bacteria: **pathogenic** (harmful) and **non-pathogenic** (harmless). Infections occur when harmful bacteria enter the skin through broken skin or hair follicles. The most common are listed below.

Boils

A boil is an infection of the hair follicle, which begins as a tender, red lump and develops into a painful pustule containing pus. It extends deep into the skin's tissue. Once a head is formed the pus is discharged, leaving a space, and so scarring of the skin often remains after the boil has healed. Poor general health and inadequate diet are factors increasing the chances of developing a boil. Sufferers are treated with antibiotics. Boils are infectious so the area affected should be avoided during massage treatment. Clients should be referred to their doctor if a boil appears on the upper lip or in the nose. Boils can be dangerous if they occur near to the eyes or the brain. **Carbuncles** are a group of boils involving several hair follicles.

Styes

A stye is a small boil on the edge of the eyelid and is caused by an infection of the follicle of an eyelash. The area becomes inflamed, swollen and there may be pus present. Styes are infectious and generally occur when a person is in poor health or has an inadequate diet.

Conjunctivitis

This is inflammation of the conjunctiva, the membrane covering the eye. The inner eyelid and eyeball appear red and sore. It is caused by a bacterial infection following irritation to the eye, such

---

Note

A **congenital condition** is a disease that is present from birth.

as grit or dust that enter the eye, and is further aggravated by rubbing. Pus is often present and may ooze from the area. Conjunctivitis is infectious and cross-infection can occur through using contaminated towels or tissues.

Impetigo

This infection begins when bacteria invade a cut, cold sore or other broken skin. It can be seen as weeping blisters that form golden/yellow-coloured crusts. The area around the crusts is inflamed and red. Impetigo is highly infectious and spreads quickly on the surface of the skin. Usually the outbreaks are among children and often go hand in hand with lice infestations. If this condition is suspected, the sufferer must be referred to a doctor and treated with antibiotics.

Folliculitis

Folliculitis is a bacterial infection of the hair follicles and sebaceous glands. The area infected is usually red and inflamed. It is infectious, so should be avoided during massage treatment.

Task 2.8

Fill in the table below.

	Brief description	Is it infectious?
Boil	....	....
Carbuncle	....	....
Conjunctivitis	....	....
Impetigo	....	....
Folliculitis	....	....

Viral infections

Although very small, **viruses** are responsible for a great deal of human disease. They are protein-coated particles of RNA or DNA. Cells in the body are taken over by invading viruses and so break down. Viruses need living cells in which to live and multiply – they cannot live outside their host. Many viruses take up residence along nerve pathways, which accounts for the pain associated with viral infections such as shingles. They can be transmitted by direct and indirect contact.

Cold sore

Cold sores are a common skin infection caused by the herpes simplex virus. It is usually passed on in early childhood, probably as a result of being kissed by someone with a cold sore. The virus passes through the skin, travels up a nerve and lies dormant at a nerve junction. When the virus is stimulated, it travels back down the nerve and forms a cold sore. It begins as an area of erythema (redness) on the skin, which blisters and forms a crust, usually around the mouth. Cold sores often appear after a period of stress. They can also be caused by exposure to bright sunlight, menstruation or accompany colds and flu. Cold sores are highly infectious so the area must be avoided during massage treatment.

Shingles

Shingles is an infection caused by the varicella zoster virus, which also causes chickenpox. It is an infection of the nerves supplying certain areas of the skin and is more common in middle-aged and older people. It appears as areas of redness and inflammation. There is itching, and blisters (sacs of fluid) develop along nerve pathways. There may be fever and lethargy too. It is a painful condition and may persist for many months. Shingles is infectious so no massage treatment should be given.

Warts

Warts are caused by a viral infection of the cells in the prickle cell layer of the skin. The cells rapidly divide in a localised area causing an irregular growth to appear above the surface of the skin. A wart is formed after hyperkeratinisation takes place and hardens the growth. Warts mainly occur on the hands and will generally disappear on their own within 2–3 years.

Plantar warts, also known as **verrucas** or verrucae, appear on the soles of the feet and grow inwards. Plantar warts are painful and can be differentiated from corns and calluses as they contain areas of black speckling and fine bleeding points. They should be removed by a doctor, although sometimes disappear by themselves. Warts and verrucas are infectious and so should not be touched.

Fill in the table below.

	Brief description	Is it infectious?
Cold sore	....	....
Shingles	....	....
Wart	....	....
Verruca	....	....

Fungal infections

Disease-causing (pathogenic) fungi produce infectious conditions. Microscopic fungi spores reproduce by the process of cell division. Fungi need other cells to survive and often affect dead tissue, such as hair and nails.

Athlete's foot (tinea pedis)

This is a common type of fungal infection. It is often transmitted in places such as saunas or swimming pools as fungi grow better in moist and warm conditions. The feet being enclosed in shoes also provide ideal conditions. It commonly affects the areas between the toes and the sole of the foot. The skin becomes cracked and itchy, with flaking pieces of dead, white skin. The skin may also become sore and swollen, and blisters form then burst. The condition is highly infectious and so the affected area must be avoided during massage treatment. Treatment of athlete's foot involves a fungicide which is applied to the toes and the shoes.

Ringworm (tinea corporis)

Ringworm is a fungal infection, not caused by a worm, and is sometimes caught through touching animals. It affects the horny layer of the skin and shows itself as red, scaly, circular patches which spread outwards. The centre of the patch heals, forming a ring shape. It usually appears on the trunk of the body, the limbs and the face. Ringworm is highly infectious so the area must be avoided during massage treatment and the client should be referred to their GP.

Fill in the table below.

	Brief description	Is it infectious?
Athlete's foot	....	....
	....	
Ringworm	....	....
	....	

Infestations

Animal parasites also cause disorders of the human skin.

Scabies

The scabies mite burrows into and lays its eggs in the horny layer of the skin. It can affect most areas of the body, although it is commonly found in the webs between the fingers and the crease of the elbow. There is a 4–6-week incubation period before the outbreak. The female mite leaves a trail of eggs and excrement in the skin, which appears as wavy greyish lines. The condition is very itchy and highly infectious. No massage treatment should be given and the client should consult their doctor.

Hair lice

This parasite lives in hair, preferably clean, and feeds off the host's blood. The female lays 4–10 eggs each day and attaches them to hair close to the scalp. This condition is itchy and so infection can occur through scratching. Specialist shampoos are available and the whole family needs to be treated. No massage treatment should be given as the condition is highly infectious.

Fill in the table below.

	Brief description	Is it infectious?
Scabies	....	....
Hair lice	....	....

Pigmentation disorders

Chloasma

This condition shows itself as patches of increased pigmentation on areas of the skin, often the face. The cause can be due to sunburn, pregnancy or the contraceptive pill. This condition is not infectious and massage treatment can be carried out.

Vitiligo

This condition shows itself as a complete loss of colour in areas of the skin. The affected areas have either lost their pigment or were never pigmented. The lightened patches of skin are very sensitive to sunlight and burn easily. The cause of vitiligo is unknown. This condition is not infectious and massage treatment can be carried out.

Albinism

In this condition, the skin and hair is abnormally white as it is unable to produce the pigment melanin. The irises of the eyes are pink. Albinism is not infectious and massage treatment can be given.

Freckles

Freckles (ephelides) show themselves as small, pigmented areas of skin. The UV rays from sunlight stimulate the production of melanin and therefore either darken freckles or create new ones. Freckles are not infectious and can be worked over during massage.

Lentigines

Lentigines (singular: lentigo) are also known as **liver spots**. Although larger than freckles, they are also pigmented areas of skin, but lentigines do not darken when exposed to UV rays. They are usually slightly raised and brown in colour and are commonly seen on the face and hands. They are not infectious and can be worked over during massage.

Naevus

A naevus (plural: naevi) is a birthmark, often found on the face or neck. It can vary in size and is usually purplish pink in colour. It is not infectious and massage can be given over the infected area.

Port wine stain

A port wine stain is a birthmark and consists of a large area of dilated capillaries, causing a reddish colour. Most occur on the head or sometimes the neck and face. They are not infectious and can be worked over during massage.

> **Note**
>
> A mole is a pigmented area of the skin and is also known as a **papilloma**.

Fill in the table below.

	Brief description	Is it infectious?
Chloasma	....	....
	....	
Vitiligo	....	....
	....	
Albinism	....	....
	....	
Freckles	....	....
	....	
Lentigo	....	....
	....	
Naevus	....	....
	....	
Port wine stain	....	....
	....	

Skin allergies

Allergies

An allergy is an abnormal response by the body's immune system to a foreign substance (**allergen**). Some people can react to ordinary substances, normally harmless to most people. Irritation to the skin causes some of its cells to release histamine, causing the skin to become warm, red and swollen.

It is advisable to give an allergy test to someone with sensitive skin; otherwise there may be a reaction to the essential oils or carrier oils. You should also ensure that the client is not allergic to wheat or nuts if you intend to use wheatgerm or carrier oils extracted from nuts. An irritated skin due to an allergy is not infectious, but it is advisable not to massage over the affected area.

Urticaria

Urticaria is an allergic skin condition often called **nettle rash** or **hives**. A red rash develops that is very itchy and disappears completely within minutes or gradually over a number of hours. There are numerous causes of urticaria; it can occur as an allergic response to substances such as certain foods and drugs. It can also be caused by heat, cold, sunlight, scabies, insect bites and contact with plants. This condition is not infectious but it is advisable not to work over the affected area during massage treatment.

Dermatitis

Dermatitis is an inflammation of the skin caused by contact with external substances. Common irritants are detergents and dyes but materials such as nylon, wool and chemicals found in perfumes can produce allergic reactions that can lead to dermatitis. Certain metals such as nickel found in watchstraps, earrings and bra hooks can irritate the skin and lead to dermatitis in sensitive people. Symptoms include erythema, itching and flaking of the skin and, in severe cases, blisters can develop. Although the condition is not infectious, it is advisable not to work over the affected area until it has cleared up.

Eczema

Eczema used to be considered to be different from dermatitis but it now generally accepted that both terms may be used to describe the same condition. Eczema is inflammation of the skin and features itchy, dry, scaly red patches. Small blisters may burst, causing the skin to weep. Hereditary factors or external irritants such as detergents, cosmetics and soaps can cause eczema. Internal irritants such as dairy products can also be a trigger. This condition is not infectious, although it is advisable to avoid working over the affected areas during massage treatment, especially if there is weeping or bleeding.

Task 2.13

Fill in the table below.

	Brief description	Is it infectious?
Allergies		
Urticaria		
Dermatitis		
Eczema		

Sebaceous gland disorders

Milia

If skin keratinises over the hair follicle it causes sebum and other substances to accumulate and become trapped in the hair follicle.

It is the keratinised skin cells that cause the hard lump. A milium (plural: milia) can be seen as a small white spot, so is often termed a **white head**, and mostly accompanies dry skin. This condition is not infectious.

Comedones

Comedones (singular: comedo), also known as **blackheads**, occur when sebum becomes trapped in a hair follicle. Keratinised cells mix with the sebum and form a plug. The head of the comedo becomes black in colour because it combines with the oxygen in the air (oxidises). Comedones generally occur on greasy skin types and are not infectious.

Acne vulgaris

Acne is a common complaint and usually affects teenagers. It is caused by an overproduction of sebum, usually due to stimulation of the sebaceous glands by hormones called testosterone and progesterone. During adolescence the levels of these sex hormones rise. The sebum, along with dead skin cells, becomes trapped in the openings of the sebaceous glands and, if they become infected, red and swollen spots will appear. Comedones (blackheads) also form and, if they become infected, the typical red and swollen spot appears. The spots are mainly found on the face, neck and back. Acne is not infectious but it is advisable for the client to consult their doctor before massage treatment.

Rosacea

This condition is often referred to as **acne rosacea**. It mainly affects people over the age of 30 and is more common in women than men. Rosacea affects the nose, cheeks and forehead, giving a flushed, reddened appearance. The blood vessels, which are dilated in these areas, produce a butterfly shape. Pus-filled spots may appear and the affected area may also become lumpy, because of swollen sebaceous glands. Causes include eating spicy or hot food,

Task 2.14

Fill in the table below.

	Brief description	Is it infectious?
Milium	....	....
Comedo	....	....
Acne vulgaris	....	....
Acne rosacea	....	....

drinking alcohol and stress. It is not an infectious condition but care needs to be taken when massaging over the affected areas. It is wise to avoid the area if the client has a severe case of rosacea.

Skin disorders involving abnormal growth

Psoriasis

In people with psoriasis, the skin cells reproduce too quickly in certain areas of the skin. This results in thickened patches of skin, which are red, dry, itchy and covered in silvery scales. Psoriasis may be mild and only affect the elbows and knees or may cover the whole body, including the scalp. The cause is unknown although the condition tends to be hereditary and stress can be a factor. Psoriasis is not infectious so massage treatment can be given providing there is no bleeding or weeping and the client will not feel any discomfort.

Skin tags

Skin tags can affect most parts of the body, often the neck. They are made of loose fibrous tissue, which protrudes out from the skin, and are mainly brown in colour. They are harmless and are not infectious. Removal of skin tags can be carried out by a doctor or certain beauty clinics. It is advisable not to work over the skin tags as it may be uncomfortable for the client.

Corns

Corns are due to thickening of the horny layer of the skin. They are the body's way of protecting itself from pressure or friction, often caused by tight or pointed shoes. Corns are commonly found on the joints of toes and can be quite painful. Corns are not infectious, but the affected area should be avoided as there may be discomfort for the client.

Skin cancer

There are three main types of skin cancer, named according to the types of skin cell from which they develop.

Basal cell carcinoma and squamous cell carcinoma

Basal cell and squamous cell carcinomas account for 95 per cent of all skin cancers. They are usually found on areas of the body often exposed to the sun, such as the face, neck, arms and hands. These cancers are often painless and begin as small, shiny, rounded lumps, which form into ulcers as they enlarge. They appear to be brought on by UV light and are usually seen in fair-skinned people. They are not infectious but should be avoided during massage treatment.

Melanoma

A melanoma is a skin growth due to overactivity of the melanocytes, usually caused by excessive exposure to the sun. Melanocyte overactivity may be benign, as in a mole, or malignant as in a malignant melanoma. Although rare and not infectious, malignant melanomas are extremely dangerous. They can occur anywhere on the body but often at the site of a mole. They are usually irregular in outline, patchy in colour, itchy or sore and may bleed. They spread very quickly and need prompt medical attention.

The danger signs to look out for are:

- any new moles that appear
- a mole that gets bigger
- a mole that bleeds, itches or ulcerates
- a mole that gets darker or lighter in colour.

Task 2.15

Fill in the table below.

	Brief description	Is it infectious?
Psoriasis	....	....
Skin tag	....	....
Corn	....	....
Basal and squamous cell carcinomas	....	....
Melanoma	....	....

HAIR

Most of the body is covered by hairs, with the exception of the palms of the hands and the soles of the feet. Hairs mainly consist of the protein keratin and grow out from **follicles**. Follicles are deep pits that extend into the dermis. Hairs help to keep the body warm and are also a form of protection. The eyelashes prevent substances from entering the eyes, and the hairs that line the nose and ears help to trap dust and bacteria.

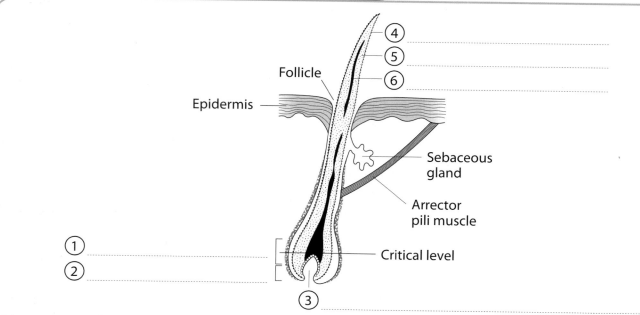

4
5
Follicle
6
Epidermis
Sebaceous gland
Arrector pili muscle
1
2
Critical level
3

Figure 2.4 *A hair and its follicle*

Label the diagram in Figure 2.4 matching the numbers to the numbered terms in the following text. Use this key to colour the diagram:

Brown – cortex (avoid the bulb area)   Red – dermal papilla.
Yellow – bulb

The ① **bulb** is found at the base of the hair and has an upper and lower part. The ② **matrix** is the lower part of the bulb and this is where cell division takes place to create the hair. When cells reach the upper part of the bulb they quickly fill with keratin and die.

Melanin can be found in the upper part of the bulb and will determine the colour of hair. The hair bulb surrounds the ③ **dermal papilla**, an area containing many blood vessels, which provides the necessary nutrients needed for hair growth.

The hair is made up of three layers:

- The ④ **cuticle** is the outer part of the hair and consists of a single layer of scale-like cells. These cells overlap rather like tiles on a roof. No pigment is contained within this layer.

Fact!

Hereditary factors will determine the specific hair growth patterns.

Fact!

Hormones are responsible for stimulating the growth of the hairs so will determine the quantity, thickness and distribution of hair on the body.

- The ⑤ **cortex** lies inside the cuticle and forms the bulk of the hair. It contains melanin, which determines the colour of the hair. The cortex helps to give strength to the hair.

- The ⑥ **medulla** is the inner part of the hair and is not always present. Air spaces in the medulla determine the colour tone and sheen of the hair because of the reflection of light.

Types of hair growth

There are different types of hair growth:

- **Lanugo hair** is the hair found on the fetus and is usually shed by about the eighth month of pregnancy.

- **Vellus hair** is soft and downy and is found all over the body except on the palms and soles of the feet.

- **Terminal hair** is longer, coarser and the follicles are deeper than vellus hair. These hairs can be found on the head, eyebrows and eyelashes, under the arms and in the pubic region.

Stages of hair growth

It takes up to seven years for the fully grown terminal hair to be shed and be replaced by a new hair. The hair grows in stages known as anagen, catagen and telogen. All hairs will be at different stages of growth at any one time.

- The **anagen** stage is the active growing stage. It lasts from a few weeks up to several years and accounts for 85 per cent of hairs at any one time. The hair bulb surrounds the nutrient-giving dermal papilla and a hair begins to grow from the matrix in the bulb. The anagen stage ends when the hair begins to separate from the dermal papilla and so no longer receives nutrients.

- **Catagen** is the transitional stage and lasts for about two weeks. Only 1 per cent of hairs will be at this stage. The hair is now fully grown and cell division has stopped. The hair has separated from the papilla and the follicle begins to shrink.

- **Telogen** is the stage at which the hair rests, and lasts for about 3–4 months. About 14 per cent of hairs will be at this stage. The resting hair will either fall out or be pushed by a new hair growing beneath it.

Fact!

The number and distribution of hair follicles are the same in both sexes.

Note

To help you remember, think of **ACT**:

A – Anagen: Active stage
C – Catagen: Changing stage
T – Telogen: Tired stage.

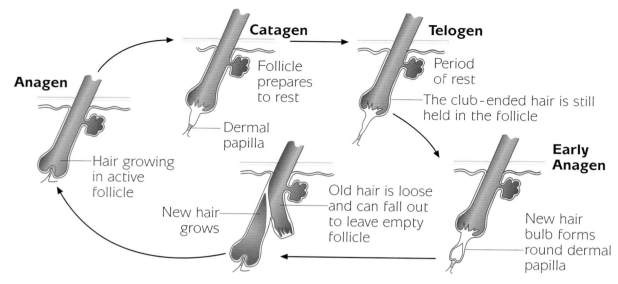

Figure 2.5 *Stages of hair growth*

Conditions associated with the hair

Alopecia

Alopecia is the term for loss of hair. **Alopecia totalis** is total hair loss from the scalp. **Alopecia areata** is a form of patchy baldness. Many women suffer from some degree of alopecia in their lives, especially after the menopause. During pregnancy scalp hair grows thicker than normal, but afterwards a decrease in hormones may cause a sudden loss of hair. Usually the loss is not noticeable because new hairs will be growing. Common reasons for hair loss include hereditary factors (which usually affect men), severe illness and stress.

Hirsutism

This is an abnormal growth of excess hair, which follows a male pattern of hair growth. It is caused by hormones called **androgens**. These hormones are made in larger amounts in men, but small amounts are also produced in women. Hirsutism can be due to an abnormally high level of androgens, or a normal level of androgens but hair follicles are oversensitive to them. Levels of androgens can increase at puberty, pregnancy, menopause and at times of stress, so all can lead to hirsutism. Hirsutism can also be caused by medical conditions such as ovarian cysts and anorexia nervosa.

Nails are formed from hard, keratinous cells and also contain some water and fat. Nails help to protect the ends of fingers and toes and are also useful for picking up small objects.

Task 2.17

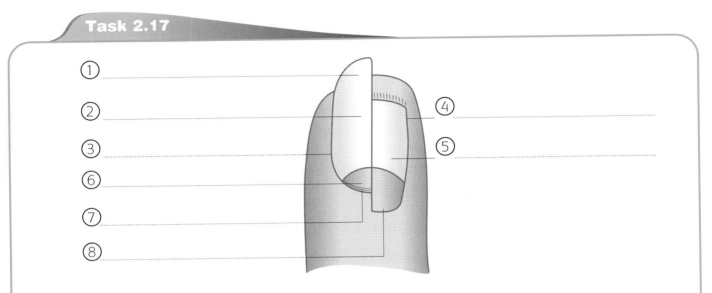

Figure 2.6 *The nail and its structures*

Label the diagram in Figure 2.6 matching the numbers to the numbered terms in the following text. Use this key to colour the diagram:

Red – nail plate
Pink – nail bed

Yellow – lunula
Blue – matrix.

① Free edge

The free edge is an extension of the nail plate and is the part that we cut and file. If you have long enough nails, look at the palm of your hand and see nail protruding over the fingertips, you will be looking at the free edge.

② Nail plate

This is the tough part of the nail that we can see. It appears pink in colour because of the blood vessels in the nail bed below it. It contains no blood vessels or nerves so can be cut without pain. Its function is to protect the nail bed beneath it.

③ Nail walls

These are overlapping folds of skin found at the side of the nails and protect the edges of the nail plate.

④ Nail grooves

Grooves at the side of the nails between the nail plate and nail wall act as guidelines for growing nails so that they grow in a straight line.

⑤ Nail bed

The nail bed is found underneath the nail plate and is rich with nerves and blood vessels. The nail bed and nail plate contain grooves and ridges which enable them to adhere perfectly with each other.

⑥ Lunula

The lunula is crescent-shaped and mostly white in colour. It is found at the base of the nail plate. It has no specific function.

⑦ Cuticle

The cuticle is the overlapping skin at the base of the nail. It prevents bacteria and any other harmful substances entering the matrix and causing infection.

⑧ Matrix

Cell division takes place in the matrix to form the nail plate. It is an area richly supplied with nerves and blood vessels. Injury to this area can mean temporary or permanent damage to the growing nail.

It takes about 5–6 months for the nail to grow from the matrix to the free edge. Diet, injury, health and age are all factors related to poor nail growth and an unhealthy appearance of the nail.

Conditions associated with the nails

The therapist needs to be aware of nail conditions that are infectious or could cause discomfort for the client during treatment. The colour of the nails is a good indication of any disorder or disease present. Nails that are yellow could indicate psoriasis, especially if there is also pitting in the nail; blue nails indicate poor circulation and if there are patches of green, brown or black there could be a fungal or bacterial infection present.

Ingrowing toenails

The side of the nail plate grows into the side of the skin at the nail wall. It can be due to ill-fitting shoes or incorrect cutting of the nail. This condition is quite painful and can lead to infection. The client should be referred to a chiropodist and the area should be avoided during treatment.

White spots

One or more white spots can be seen on the nail plate. They are due to minor injury to the base of the nail – a tiny air pocket forms between the nail bed and nail plate. They may also be a sign of zinc deficency in the diet. This condition is not infectious and treatment can be given.

Fungal nail infection

A fungal nail infection is caused by the same fungus that causes athlete's foot so a third of people with this condition will eventually develop a fungus of the nail. The fungus normally attacks the nail from the free edge or the side of the nail and spreads slowly towards the cuticle. The nail changes to a yellow or creamy colour and may begin to thicken and crumble. Sometimes the end of the nail may separate from the nail bed. The client needs to be referred to the doctor and the affected area should be avoided.

Paronychia

Paronychia (pa-ro-nic-ee-ah) is an infection of the skin down the side of the nail. The skin becomes damaged and bacteria enter and cause an infection. This condition is often painful and can be unsightly as pus may build up around the nail. If the condition lasts for more than two weeks there may be a fungal rather than bacterial infection. Bacterial infections are treated with antibiotics and fungal infections are treated with fungal creams. It is obviously wise to avoid the affected nail during treatment.

Pterygium

Pterygium (te-rij-ee-um) features thick, hard, overgrown cuticles that adhere to the nail plate. Splitting of the cuticle may result, which could lead to infection. It is due to neglect of the nails. It is not infectious so treatment can be given.

Fill in the table below.

	Brief description	Should area be avoided during treatment?
Ingrowing toenail	....	....
White spots	....	....
Fungal nail infection	....	....
Paronychia	....	....
Pterygium	....	....

The skeletal system

There are 206 bones in the adult body.

The skeletal system consists of the bones and joints of the body. There are 206 bones in the body, which continue to grow up to the age of 18–25. After 25 the bones stop growing, although they can still continue to thicken.

Bone is living tissue and is constantly being built up and broken down. It is the hardest of all connective tissue in the body. It is made up of 30 per cent living tissue and 70 per cent minerals and water. The minerals include mainly calcium and phosphorus.

FUNCTIONS OF THE SKELETON

Note

To help you remember the functions, think of **SAD PAM**.

- **S – Shape/support** The skeleton gives the body its shape and supports the weight of all the other tissues.
- **A – Attachment for muscles and tendons** Bones provide the attachment point for the tendons of most skeletal muscles.
- **D – Development of blood cells** Red blood cells, white blood cells and platelets are produced within the red bone marrow of the bone.
- **P – Protection** Bones help to protect vital organs from injury; for example, the ribs protect the heart and lungs and the skull protects the brain.
- **A – Allows movements of the body** When skeletal muscles contract, they pull on bones to produce a movement.
- **M – Mineral store** Bones store the minerals calcium and phosphorus, which are important for the strength of the bone. If these minerals are required elsewhere in the body, the bones can release them into the bloodstream.

BONES

Fact!

99 per cent of calcium is found in the bones and teeth. However, the remaining 1 per cent is very important and its uses include muscle contraction and the passing of nerve messages in the body.

Formation of bone

The formation of bone is known as **ossification** and continually happens throughout life. It is more active during the period of body growth and following the fracture of a bone.

In the developing embryo, rods of cartilage covered by a membrane can be seen and will eventually become the long bones. Bone-making cells called **osteoblasts** produce minerals and collagen. They first manufacture bone in the middle of the cartilage which eventually becomes the shaft of the long bone.

The membrane becomes the **periosteum** and bone and mineral salts are laid down. This results in an increase of thickness and length of the bone. Cells known as **osteoclasts** break down areas within the bone. A cavity is formed which will become filled with red bone marrow. Usually at the time of birth, bone is produced at each end of the cartilage and will extend towards the shaft. A thin layer of cartilage will remain to cover each end of the bone.

Bone tissue

There are two types of bone tissue called compact and cancellous (spongy).

Compact bone tissue

Compact bone tissue is hard and dense. It provides strength, support and protection. It forms the outer layer of all bones and most of the shaft of long bones such as the thigh bone (femur). Under a microscope, compact bone looks like honeycomb and many circles can be seen, known as **Haversian** (ha-ver-shan) **systems**. In the centre of these circles are channels running lengthways through the bone called the **Haversian canals**. The Haversian canals contain nerves, lymph capillaries and blood vessels.

The **lamellae** are rings of bone consisting of mineral salts (mostly

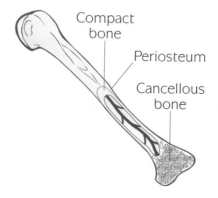

Figure 3.1 *Compact and cancellous bone*

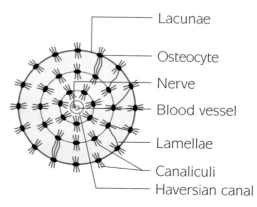

Figure 3.2 *Haversian system in compact bone*

Note

Think of the **cell** in can**cell**ous to help you remember that red blood cells are made in the marrow of cancellous bone.

Fact!

Red bone marrow produces billions of red blood cells every day in adults.

calcium phosphates), which gives the bone its hardness. Rope-like collagen fibres give the bone its strength. The **lacunae** are the small spaces between the lamellae and contain the bone-making cells called **osteocytes** (fully grown osteoblasts). Narrow canals called **canaliculi** radiate from the lacunae. The canaliculi are filled with tissue fluid containing oxygen and nutrients for the bone tissue.

Cancellous bone tissue

Cancellous bone has a spongy appearance and so is often called **spongy bone**. The spongy bone helps to give great strength but also keeps the skeleton light. Spongy bone is found in the end of long bones and in short, flat and irregularly shaped bones. The cancellous bone is filled with red bone marrow. Red bone marrow produces billions of red blood cells every day in adults.

Types of bone

Almost all bones except the coccyx (tail bone) are designed to meet a particular need in the body. There are five main types of bone:

- **Long bones**, such as the humerus in the arm, have a long shaft and two wider ends. They act as levers to enable the body to move. Other examples of long bones include the femur (thigh bone), tibia, fibula (both found in the lower leg), radius, ulna (both found in the lower arm) metacarpals (in the hand) and phalanges (found in fingers and toes).

- **Short bones** are roughly cube-shaped. They are found where strength rather than mobility is required. Bones of the wrists (carpals) and ankles (tarsals) are examples of short bones.

- **Flat bones** help to protect vital organs in the body. Flat bones such as the skull protect the brain and the ribs protect the heart and lungs. Other flat bones include the scapulae (shoulder blades) and the sternum (breast bone).

- **Irregular bones** such as the vertebrae of the spine (backbones) are found in places where extra strength is needed and also make good attachment points for muscles.

- **Sesamoid bones** are small rounded bones that develop in the tendons. They enable the tendon to move smoothly over certain bones. An example is the patella (knee cap), which prevents wear and tear on the tendon of the front thigh muscle, which is attached to the tibia. It keeps the tendon in place when the knee is bent. They are also found in the palms of the hands and soles of the feet. For example, these bones can be found in tendons lying over the joint, under the head of the first metatarsal in the foot. Their purpose is to protect the tendon as it moves over the joint. They may vary in number from person to person and mostly measure only a few millimetres.

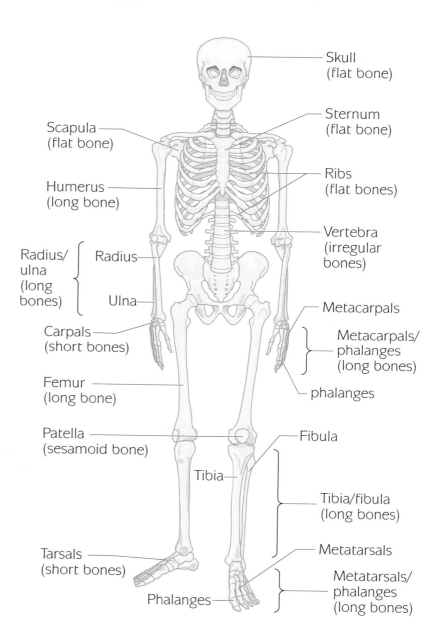

Figure 3.3 *Types of bone*

Which types of bones are the following and what are their functions?

Type of bone	Function
Carpals	....
Vertebrae	....
Humerus	....
Skull	....

Fact!

Regular exercise is essential – not only does it prevent loss of bone but it also stimulates the formation of new, stronger bone tissue. Bones adapt to the stress of exercise by laying down more calcium and other minerals and also increase the amount of collagen fibres.

Condition associated with bones

Osteoporosis

Bones are living tissue and so are constantly changing, losing and gaining protein and calcium to and from the blood stream. Bones are naturally being built up and broken down. **Osteoporosis** causes the bone to break down faster than it is being formed. This causes the bones to become porous and thin and so there is an increased risk of fracture.

It mainly affects middle-aged and older people and is more common in women than men. Hormones such as oestrogen in women and testosterone in men help stimulate the bone-forming cells, oesteoblasts, to produce new bone tissue. Women produce smaller amounts of oestrogen after the menopause, and men produce smaller amounts of testosterone as they age. As a result the osteoblasts become less active, and there is a decrease in bone mass.

A well-balanced diet, which includes plenty of vitamin D and calcium, as well as exercise, can help protect against osteoporosis later in life.

LIGAMENTS

Ligaments consist of bands of strong, fibrous connective tissue which are silvery in appearance. They prevent dislocation by holding the bones together across joints but stretch slightly to allow movement. When excess strain is put on a joint, especially the ankle or knee, the ligaments can become sprained or torn. Injuries to ligaments can be minor or severe, and result in bruising, tenderness and swelling. Minor injury can be treated with ice packs to reduce the swelling and then bandaged to support the joint. As ligaments have a relatively poor blood supply when damaged, they can take a long time to heal.

TENDONS

Tendons consist of white, strong, almost inelastic, fibrous bands. Most muscles are attached to bones by tendons. They vary in length and thickness. When a muscle contracts, the force transmitted through the tendon creates movement at the bone. An example of a tendon is the achilles tendon that attaches from the calf muscle to the back of the foot.

A tendon can become injured if stretched beyond its limit. This happens in twisted ankles and sprained wrists as the bodyweight is suddenly concentrated in one small area putting strain on the tendon. The tendon may partially tear when some fibres are torn. The remaining intact fibres hold the torn ends in contact so, with rest, the ends reunite and the area heals. There can also be a complete tearing in which the tendon is severed. The tendon can tear away from the bone or muscle and this is extremely painful.

Condition associated with tendons

Tennis elbow

Tennis elbow is a painful condition in which there is inflammation of the tendon that attaches the muscle of the forearm to the bone of the upper arm. The sufferer will feel discomfort if the elbow is straightened. It can be caused by wrenching, or the overuse of muscles, such as when playing tennis or weight-lifting. It also affects people whose work involves activities such as lifting or using tools.

> **Fact!**
>
> Remember:
>
> - **Ligaments** attach bone to bone.
> - **Tendons** attach muscle to bone.

ANATOMICAL TERMS

To understand these terms the body has to be viewed in the correct anatomical position. The body stands erect with arms by the side and palms facing forwards. There is an imaginary vertical line that runs through the middle of the body and is known as the **midline** (see Figure 3.15).

- **Medial** – nearer to the midline of the body. The ulna is on the medial side of the forearm. The inside of the leg and foot is the medial side.

- **Lateral** – towards the outer side or further away from the midline of the body. The humerus is lateral to the clavicle. The outside of the leg and foot is the lateral side.

- **Anterior or ventral** – nearer to or at the front of the body. The sternum is anterior to the heart.

- **Posterior or dorsal** – nearer to or at the back of the body. The heart is posterior to the sternum. The top of the foot is the dorsal surface.

- **Plantar** – on or towards the sole of the foot.

- **Proximal** – closer to the midline. In the limbs it is the part nearer to the trunk. The humerus is proximal to the radius.

- **Distal** – further away from the midline. In the limbs it is the part that is further away from the trunk. The phalanges are distal to the carpals.

- **Superficial** – towards the surface of the body. The skin is superficial to the heart.

- **Deep** – away from the surface of the body. The heart is deep to the skin.

THE BONES OF THE SKELETON

Bones of the skull and face

① **Frontal bone** One frontal bone forms the forehead.

② **Parietal** (pa-ri'e-tal) **bone** Two parietal bones form the sides and top of the skull.

③ **Temporal bone** Two temporal bones are found at the sides of the skull under the parietals.

④ **Occipital bone** One occipital bone forms the back of the skull.

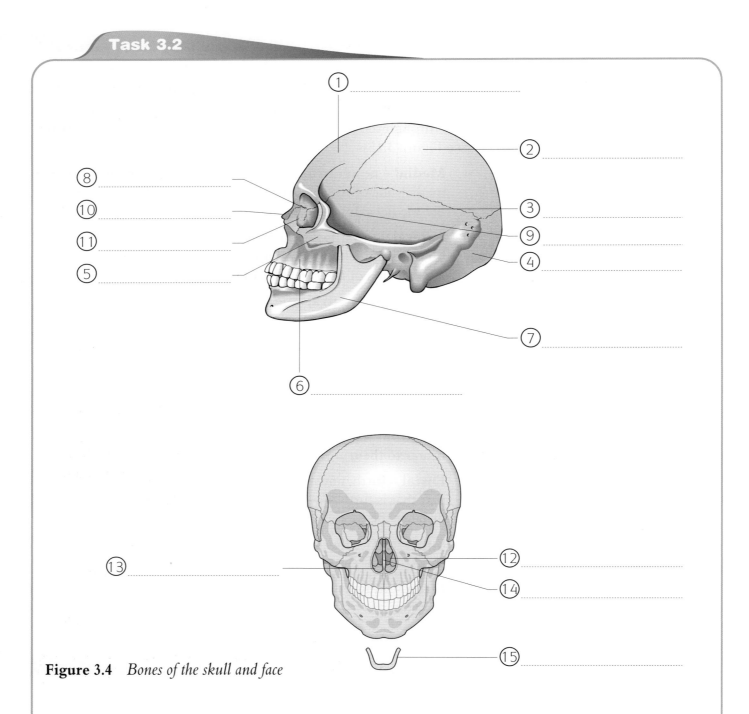

Figure 3.4 *Bones of the skull and face*

Label the diagram in Figure 3.4 using the information on pages 51 and 53. Use this key to colour the diagram:

Blue – frontal and occipital bones
Yellow – parietal and nasal bones
Green – temporal and ethmoid bones
Red – mandible and palatine

Orange – maxilla and sphenoid
Purple – lacrimal and hyoid
Grey – turbinator and vomer
Pink – zygomatic bones.

⑤ **Zygomatic bone** Two zygomatic bones form the cheekbones.

⑥ **Maxilla** The maxilla forms the upper part of the jaw.

⑦ **Mandible** The mandible forms the lower part of the jaw. It is the only movable bone of the skull.

⑧ **Ethmoid** One ethmoid bone helps to form the eye socket and nasal cavities.

⑨ **Sphenoid** (sfee'noid) One sphenoid bone helps to form the base of the skull.

⑩ **Nasal** Two nasal bones form the bridge of the nose.

⑪ **Lacrimal bone** Two lacrimal bones make up part of each eye socket.

⑫ **Turbinates** Two turbinated bones make up part of the nasal cavity.

⑬ **Palatine bones** Two L-shaped palatine bones form the walls of the nasal cavities and part of the roof of the mouth.

⑭ **Vomer** One vomer extends upwards from the hard palate to make the nasal septum.

⑮ **Hyoid** One horseshoe-shaped bone lying in the neck. It is not joined to any other bone. However, it is attached to the temporal bone by ligaments.

Bones of the shoulder girdle

① **Clavicle** – a long slender bone also known as the collar bone.

② **Scapula** (plural – scapulae) – a large, triangular, flat bone also known as the shoulder blade.

Bones of the thorax

The thoracic cavity contains organs such as the heart and lungs, which are protected by the ribcage.

③ **Ribs** There are 12 pairs of ribs.

④ **Sternum** Also known as the breast bone.

Bones of the upper limbs

⑤ **Humerus** The long bone of the upper arm.

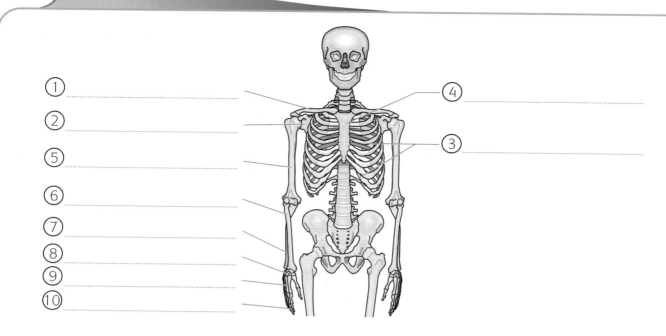

Figure 3.5 *Bones of the upper body*

Label the diagram in Figure 3.5 using the information on pages 53–4. Use this key to colour the diagram:

Yellow – clavicle
Blue – scapula (see also Figure 4.6)
Pink – humerus
Red – ulna

Green – radius
Orange – carpals, metacarpals and phalanges
Brown – sternum
Purple – ribs.

Note

- The **axial skeleton** is made up of the skull, spine, ribs and sternum.

- The **appendicular skeleton** is made up of the shoulder girdle, arms and hands, the pelvic bones and the legs and feet.

⑥ **Radius** The bone situated on the thumb side of the forearm.

⑦ **Ulna** The bone situated on the little-finger side of the forearm.

⑧ The **carpals** consist of eight small bones in each wrist (see Figure 3.6).

⑨ The **metacarpals** consist of five metacarpal bones (long bones), which form the palm of each hand.

⑩ There are 14 **phalanges** in each hand, three in each finger and two in the thumb.

Bones of the hand and wrist

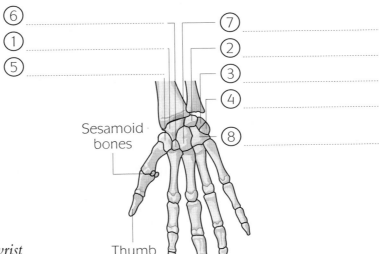

Figure 3.6 *Bones of the hand and wrist*

Label the diagram in Figure 3.6 using the information below. Use this key to colour the diagram:

Blue – scaphoid and trapezium
Red – lunate and trapezoid
Brown – hamate and triquetral

Green – pisiform and capitate
Yellow – phalanges
Orange – metacarpals.

Note

To help you remember the bones of the hands think of the following three words, but remember to drop the vowels: 'to touch plates'.

The carpals are: ① **scaphoid**, ② **lunate**, ③ **triquetral**, ④ **pisiform**, ⑤ **trapezium**, ⑥ **trapezoid**, ⑦ **capitate**, ⑧ **hamate**.

They are closely fitted together and held in position by ligaments. Tendons of muscles in the forearm cross over the wrist joint, and are held close to these bones by strong fibrous bands called **retinacula**.

Bones of the pelvic girdle

The pelvic girdle consists of three bones fused together:

① The **ilium** is the largest of the three bones. The iliac crest can be felt by placing the hand on the hip.

② The **ischium** (iss'kee-um) forms the posterior aspect of the pelvis.

③ The **pubis** is situated on the anterior aspect of the pelvis. The female's pelvis is wider and shallower and so has more space than the male's. This is due to the requirements of pregnancy and childbirth.

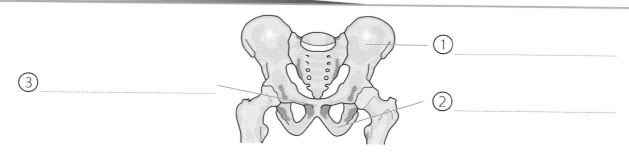

Figure 3.7 *The pelvic girdle*

Label the diagram in Figure 3.7 using the information on page 55. Use this key to colour the diagram:

Red – ilium
Brown – pubis

Orange – ischium.

Bones of the lower limbs

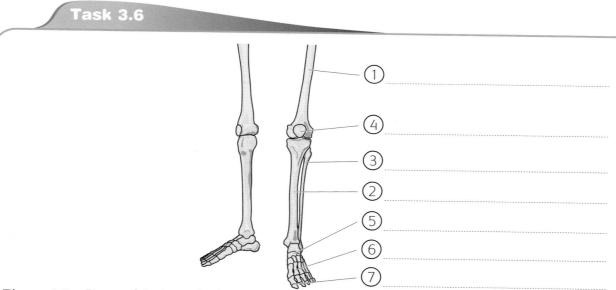

Figure 3.8 *Bones of the lower limbs*

Label the diagram in Figure 3.8 using the information on page 57. Use this key to colour the diagram:

Red – femur
Orange – patella
Blue – tibia

Yellow – fibula
Green – tarsals, metatarsals and phalanges.

Note

To remember that carpals are found in the wrist and tarsals below in the ankle, think of **CAR on the TAR**.

① **Femur** The thigh bone, the longest bone in the body.

② **Tibia** The bone situated on the anterior aspect of the lower leg, also known as the shin bone.

③ **Fibula** The bone situated on the lateral side of the tibia and thinner than the tibia.

④ **Patella** The knee cap, which articulates with the femur.

⑤ **Tarsals** The seven bones of the ankle.

⑥ **Metatarsals** There are five metatarsal bones in each foot.

⑦ **Phalanges** There are 14 phalanges in each foot and these form the toes.

Bones of the vertebral column (spine)

Task 3.7

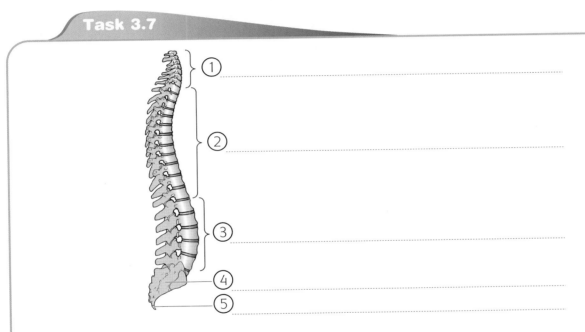

Figure 3.9 *Bones of the vertebral column*

Label the diagram in Figure 3.9 using the information on page 58. Use this key to colour the diagram:

Yellow – cervical spine
Green – thoracic spine
Blue – lumbar region

Orange – sacrum
Red – coccyx.

The vertebral column supports the upper body and encloses and protects the spinal cord. It consists of 33 bones which are divided into five groups: cervical, thoracic, lumbar, sacral and coccygeal:

Note

- The 1st cervical vertebra is a ring of bone known as the **atlas**.
- The 2nd vertebra is known as the **axis**.

① The **cervical spine** consists of seven vertebrae.

② The **thoracic spine** consists of 12 vertebrae.

③ The **lumbar spine** consists of five bones which are the largest vertebrae.

④ The **sacrum** consists of five vertebrae fused together.

⑤ The **coccyx** consists of four bones fused together.

In total: 33 bones.

Note

The **sacroiliac joint** is the joint found between the sacrum and the ilium (hip bone).

Intervertebral discs

Between the bones of the spine are pads of white fibrocartilage known as **intervertebral discs**. The intervertebral discs are thicker in the lumbar region than in the cervical region and are kept in place by ligaments. Their functions are to act as shock absorbers and to give the spine some flexibility so movement can take place.

Bones and arches of the feet

Task 3.8

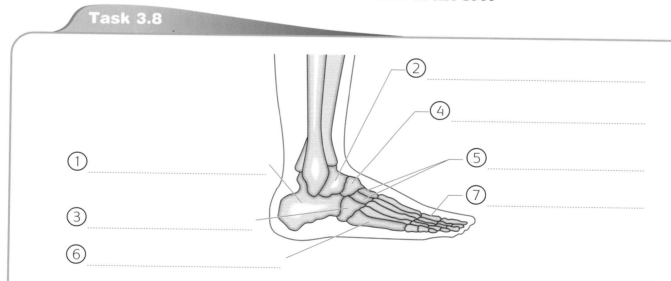

Figure 3.10 *Bones of the feet*

Label the diagram in Figure 3.10 using the information on page 59. Use this key to colour the diagram:

Green – calcaneus
Red – talus
Blue – cuboid
Brown – navicular

Orange – cuneiforms
Pink – metatarsals
Yellow – phalanges.

The bones of the feet make up a bridge-like structure. There are seven tarsal (ankle) bones, which form the posterior part of the foot:

① **calcaneus** (kal-kay'nee-us) – one

② **talus** – one

③ **cuboid** – one

④ **navicular** – one

⑤ **cuneiforms** – three

⑥ **metatarsals** – five

⑦ **phalanges** – 14, which form the toes.

Arches of the foot

The bones of the feet fit together to make arches. The arches help to support the weight of the body and provide leverage when walking. Strong ligaments and tendons support the bones that form the arches.

Task 3.9

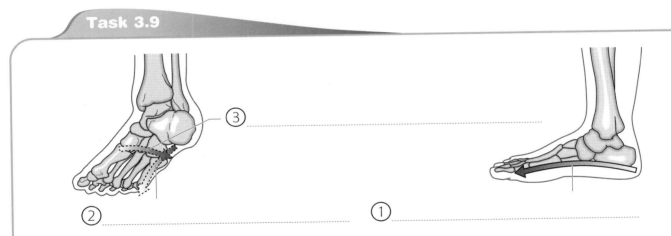

Figure 3.11 *Arches of the foot*

Label the diagram in Figure 3.11 using the information below and on page 60. Use this key to colour the diagram:

Red – medial longitudinal arch
Blue – lateral longitudinal arch

Green – transverse arch.

The arches of the foot are:

① The **medial longitudinal arch** is the highest arch on the big-toe side of the foot. It begins at the calcaneum, rises to the talus and descends through the navicular, the three cuneiforms and the three medial metatarsals.

② The **lateral longitudinal arch** is on the little-toe side of the foot and begins at the calcaneum. It rises at the cuboid and descends to the two outer metatarsal bones.

③ The **transverse arch** runs between the medial and lateral aspect of the foot and is formed by the navicular, the cuneiform bones and the bases of the five metatarsals.

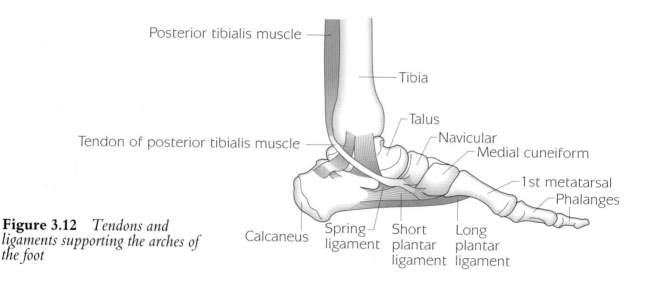

Figure 3.12 *Tendons and ligaments supporting the arches of the foot*

Posterior tibialis muscle

Tibia

Tendon of posterior tibialis muscle

Talus
Navicular
Medial cuneiform
1st metatarsal
Phalanges

Calcaneus
Spring ligament
Short plantar ligament
Long plantar ligament

Conditions associated with the arches of the foot

Flatfoot
Weakening of the ligaments and tendons that hold the arches in place can cause the medial longitudinal arch to flatten and the result is flatfoot. The causes include injuries to the foot and ankle, excessive weight, hereditary factors or a postural abnormality.

Clawfoot
In this condition the medial longitudinal arch is too high. Muscle deformities can cause clawfoot and it is occasionally found in diabetics where the muscles of the foot have wasted away.

Clubfoot
This is an inherited condition in which the feet are malformed. The foot twists in an inward and downwards direction and there is an increase in the angle of the arch. Corrective action may involve surgery, corrective shoes or applying casts soon after birth.

Bunions

Bunions can be due to weaknesses in the arches of the feet. Ill-fitting shoes worn over a long period of time can cause bunions. The large joint at the base of the big toe sticks out and so forces the big toes inwards towards the other toes.

JOINTS OF THE BODY

'A joint' describes the joining (articulation) of two or more bones of the body. There are three main types of joint:

- **Fibrous** or **immovable joints** are fixed joints in which no movement between the joints is possible. Examples are the sutures or joints between the skull bones.

- **Cartilaginous joints** are slightly movable joints in which only limited movement is possible. Examples are the joints between the bones of the vertebral column, with their intervertebral discs of fibrocartilage.

- **Synovial joints** are freely movable joints, of which there are several types, all having similar characteristics. An example is the joint of the knee.

Synovial joints

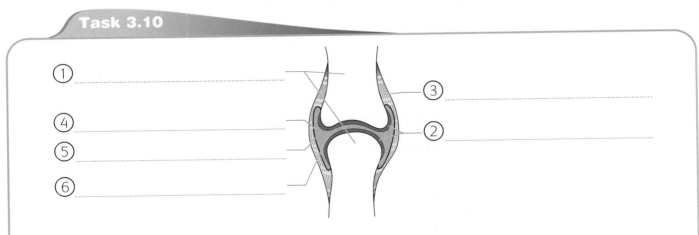

Task 3.10

Figure 3.13 *Structure of a synovial joint*

Label the diagram in Figure 3.13 using the information on page 62. Use this key to colour the diagram:

Yellow – bones
Green – ligaments

Blue – hyaline cartilage
Orange – joint cavity and synovial fluid.

In a freely movable joint ends of the ① **bones** are mostly covered by ② **hyaline cartilage**. The cartilage helps to reduce friction and acts as a shock absorber during movement. ③ **Ligaments** are needed to bind the bones together and help prevent dislocation. The space between the bones is called the ④ **joint cavity** and is enclosed by a capsule of fibrous tissue. The ⑤ **synovial membrane** lines the joint cavity and secretes a fluid called ⑥ **synovial fluid**, which lubricates the joint and provides the hyaline cartilage with nutrients.

There are various types of synovial joint (see Figure 3.14).

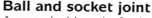

Ball and socket joint

A rounded head of a bone fits into a cup-shaped cavity permitting movements in all planes. Movements possible are flexion, extension, adduction, abduction, rotation and circumduction.
Examples are the shoulder and hip joints.

Hinge joint

A round surface fits into the hollow surface of another bone, permitting movement in one plane only.
Examples are the elbow and knee joints.

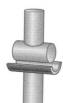

Saddle joint

Similar to a hinge joint, but allows more movement. Movements possible are flexion, extension, abduction, adduction and slight circumduction.
Examples include the joint between the thumb and carpals and the joint between the skull and lower jaw.

Condyloid joint

Condyloid joints allow movement in two planes.
An example is the wrist.

Pivot joint

A socket in one bone rotates around a peg on another, therefore a rotation movement is possible.
An example is the first cervical vertebra, which rotates around the second to turn the head.

Gliding joint

Two flat surfaces of bone glide over each other to make back-and-forth and side-to-side movements.
Examples are the joints between the carpals and tarsals.

Figure 3.14 *Types of synovial joint*

State whether the following synovial joints are ball and socket, hinge, saddle, pivot or gliding joints.

Joint	Type
Hip	....
First and second vertebra	....
Elbow	....
Between tarsals	....
Knee	....
Shoulder	....
Between carpals	....
Between skull and lower jaw	....

Joint movements

Joints allow several different types of movement to be made (Figure 3.15). There are some basic terms used to describe these movements:

- **flexion** – a movement in which the body part bends and there is a decrease in the angle between the articulating bones

- **extension** – the opposite of flexion: the angle between the articulating bones increases and the body part straightens

- **adduction** – movement towards the midline of the body

- **abduction** – movement away from the midline of the body

- **rotation** – the rotary movement of bone around its axis

- **circumduction** – a circular movement

- **supination** – rotating the forearm, turning the palm of the hand to face outwards

- **pronation** – rotating the forearm, turning the palm to face inwards

- **inversion** – inward movement of the foot towards the medial line

- **eversion** – outward movement of the foot away from the medial line.

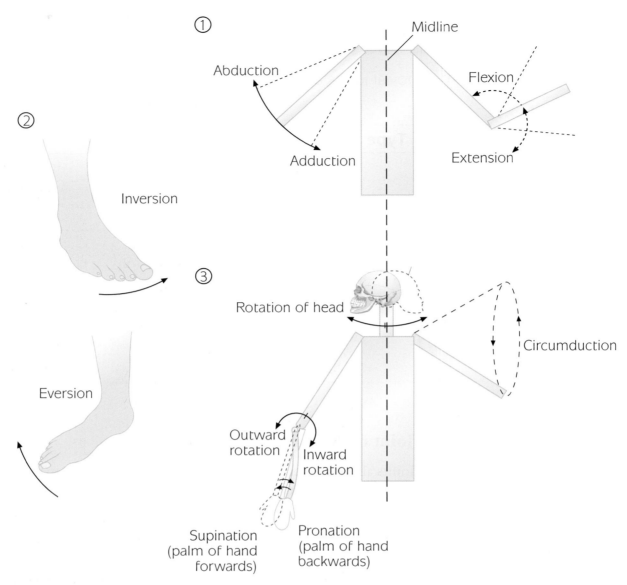

Figure 3.15 *Joint movements*

Conditions associated with joints

Bursitis

Some synovial joints contain a sac-like structure called a bursa, which helps to provide padding where tendons rub against bones or other tendons. Bursitis is inflammation of the bursa which may be due to injury or repetitive stress. Examples include tennis elbow and housemaid's knee.

Sprain

A sprain can be caused by wrenching or twisting a joint, causing injury to its ligaments. It occurs when ligaments are stressed beyond their normal capacity.

Arthritis

The term 'arthritis' refers to many different diseases, most of which are characterised by inflammation of one or more joints. Pain and stiffness may also be present in muscles near the joint. The two main kinds are osteoarthritis and rheumatoid arthritis.

- **Osteoarthritis** is the most common form of arthritis, which one in ten people will suffer from. Wear and tear on the joint will cause the cartilage to become damaged and so it literally wears away. Osteoarthritis is more common in people who regularly take part in vigorous exercise. It causes pain and restricted movement, and particularly affects movable joints that tend to be weight-bearing, such as the knees and hips.

- **Rheumatoid arthritis** is the more severe form of arthritis and will affect one person in a hundred. It is more common in females and can affect all ages. It is a condition where the body attacks its own tissues and is therefore known as an **autoimmune disease**. The membrane that lines the joint becomes completely swollen. The cause may be viral infection or hereditary factors. There will be inflammation and swelling around the joints. There may also be pain and loss of function. It mostly affects the joints of the hands and feet.

Gout

Gout is a disease of the joints in which uric acid crystals build up around joints, tendons and other tissues of the body. Crystals form when the levels of uric acid in the body are abnormally high. Gout usually begins with pain and inflammation in the joint of the big toe.

Frozen shoulder

This is inflammation of the shoulder joint which may be a result of muscle injury. There is inflammation and thickening of the lining of the capsule in which the shoulder is held. It causes pain and stiffness around the shoulder and movement becomes increasingly difficult.

Fractures

When a bone breaks it is called a fracture. There are different types of fracture:

- A **simple fracture** occurs if the bone breaks but the skin remains intact and the tissue around it is not broken.

- A **compound fracture** means the broken ends of the bone protrude through the skin.

- A **comminuted fracture** occurs if the bone breaks in two or more places.

- An **impacted fracture** is when part of a broken bone impacts into another.

- A **greenstick fracture** is a partial fracture, occurring only in children as their bones are soft; when stress is placed on the bone, one side of it may bend enough to cause the other side to splinter.

Muscles

4

There are over 600 muscles in the body, which make up 40–50 per cent of the body weight. The function of the muscles is to produce movement, maintain posture and provide heat for the body.

The muscular system consists of three types of muscle:

- **Involuntary muscle** is also known as **smooth muscle**. Such muscles are involuntary because they are not under our conscious control. The cells of the muscles are spindle-shaped. Smooth muscle makes up the walls of the blood and lymph vessels, along with other vessels. The muscles allow the walls to relax and constrict.

- The **cardiac muscle** is specialised tissue found only in the heart. This muscle never tires; if it did we would have serious problems! Even if the heart is separated from the body, it will continue to beat for a while.

- Therapists are mostly concerned with **voluntary muscles**, which are under our conscious control and are also known as the **skeletal muscles**. Skeletal muscles consist of bundles of muscle fibres, striped in appearance and enclosed in a sheath (fascia). They allow movement of the body.

Fact!

There are over 600 muscles in the body.

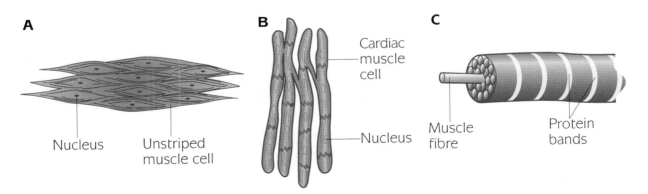

Figure 4.1 *Types of muscle: A Involuntary (smooth muscle); B Cardiac muscle; C Voluntary (skeletal) muscle*

Muscle contraction

Skeletal muscle tissue consists of bundles of long, thin muscle fibres. Inside each fibre are thread-like **myofibrils**, which extend the entire length of the muscle fibre. Myofibrils contain two types of overlapping protein called filaments, which lie side by side. They do not extend the whole length of the muscle fibre but are arranged into sections. The thinner filaments are called **actin**, and the thicker filaments are known as **myosin**. The overlapping of these filaments gives muscle fibres their striped appearance (Figure 4.2). When a muscle contracts, it shortens and thickens. This is because the thinner filaments (actin) slide in between the thicker filaments (myosin). When the muscle relaxes the thinner filaments slide back out again (Figure 4.3).

> **Fact!**
>
> 80,000 myosin filaments laid side-by-side would only be 1 mm wide.

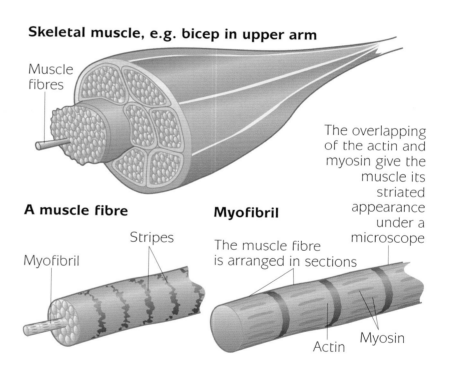

Skeletal muscle, e.g. bicep in upper arm

Muscle fibres

The overlapping of the actin and myosin give the muscle its striated appearance under a microscope

A muscle fibre

Myofibril

Stripes

Myofibril

The muscle fibre is arranged in sections

Actin

Myosin

Figure 4.2 *The interior of a muscle*

Skeletal muscles are richly supplied with blood vessels and nerves. Before movement of a muscle can occur, a message must be sent from the brain through a motor nerve, which in turn stimulates the muscle to contract. The point at which a motor nerve enters a muscle is called the **motor point**. A motor nerve branches out, the ends of which are called **motor end plates**, and rest on muscle fibres. Each muscle fibre has its

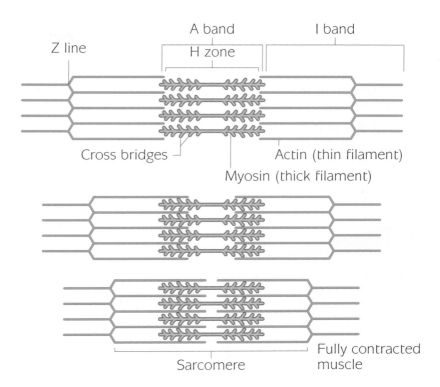

Z line

A band

I band

H zone

Cross bridges

Actin (thin filament)

Myosin (thick filament)

Sarcomere

Fully contracted muscle

Figure 4.3 *The mechanism of contraction of a muscle*

own nerve ending. Branches of one motor nerve can stimulate up to 150 muscle fibres at any one time.

Skeletal muscles bring about movement by exerting a pull on tendons, which cause the bones to move at the joints. The pulling force that causes movement is due to contraction (shortening) of the muscle.

Fascia

Muscles are covered in fibrous tissue called **fascia** (fash'-ee-ah). This sheath extends to become **tendons** and attaches the muscle to bone. Fascia allows the muscles to glide smoothly past each other but they sometimes adhere to each other. Then the affected muscles do not function as well, so there may be restricted movement and some discomfort.

Muscle tone

Muscle is never completely at rest but in a state of partial contraction. The partial contraction is not enough to move the muscle but will cause some tension. All skeletal muscles must be slightly contracted if the body is to remain upright. If all of the muscles relaxed, the body would fall to the floor. This continuous slight tension is involuntary and is known as **muscle tone**.

Fact!

- **Atony** refers to a low amount of, or lack of, muscle tone.
- Poor diet or lack of use can cause muscles to **atrophy** (waste away).

Note

Oxygen debt is when oxygen supplies have been used up, such as during vigorous exercise, and oxygen cannot be supplied fast enough to the muscle fibres. Breathing is increased to help repay the oxygen debt.

Fact!

Vigorous exercise can cause minor tearing of muscle fibres and is thought to be a major reason why muscles become sore and stiff 12–48 hours afterwards.

Different groups of muscle fibres contract at different times; this prevents the muscle from becoming fatigued.

Each person's degree of muscle tone varies depending on the amount of activity or exercise taken. People who are sedentary and do not exercise usually have poor muscle tone as the muscle fibres do not contract as far as they should. This results in a lowering of muscle tone and so the muscles are said to be **flaccid**. Muscles with a high degree of tone are called **spastic** as they are hard and rigid as a result of over-contraction. This can be seen in body-builders. Regular exercise and massage can help to maintain the elasticity of the muscle fibres, which will improve the tone of the muscle.

Muscle fatigue

Muscles require fuel in the form of glucose, and oxygen is needed to burn the glucose to make energy. When muscles become overworked, for example during vigorous exercise, the oxygen and glucose supplies are used up. If there is insufficient oxygen and glucose, the muscles cannot produce enough energy to contract. The contractions will be become weaker until they eventually stop. This is known as **muscle fatigue**.

As a result, an accumulation of harmful waste products such as lactic acid and carbon dioxide starts to build up in the affected muscle, causing stiffness and pain. Muscle fatigue is common among athletes who compete in endurance sports such as marathon races. Resting and gentle massage of the muscle will ensure that the blood brings oxygen and glucose and removes the waste products so that the muscles can work properly again.

Conditions associated with muscles

Muscle strain

Overwork or overstretching of the muscles can cause **strain** and may result in muscle fibres being torn. It can normally be felt as hardness in the muscle, usually running in the same direction as the muscle fibres.

Tearing of muscle fibres

Injury to a muscle can cause complete or partial tearing of the muscle fibres. Partial tears result in the tearing of some muscle fibres and will feel very tender and painful, especially when contracting the muscle. Complete tearing involves tearing of all the muscle fibres, which causes the two ends of the muscles to contract away from each other. It is extremely painful and there is complete loss of function.

Adhesions and fibrous tissue

Injury and damage to the muscle may cause scar tissue to form due to insufficient healing by collagen fibres. This may be due to the fact the muscles remained tense while healing took place. The scar tissue creates adhesions and fibrous tissue. Muscle fibres need to be able to glide smoothly past each other but cannot do this when the fibres are stuck together (**adhesions**). After a while the fibres will knit together and form a hard lump or knot (**fibrous tissue**).

Cramp

Cramp is a painful muscle spasm that may arise following exercise. Muscle spasms occur when muscles contract for too long, or when excessive sweating causes water and salt loss. The accumulation of lactic acid in the muscles following vigorous exercise may also cause cramp. Lightly massaging and gradually stretching the affected muscle can relieve the spasm and pain. Sometimes cramp can occur for no reason, for example during sleep, and may be due to poor muscle tone.

Fibrositis

This is a common muscular condition in which there is a build-up of urea and lactic acid inside the muscle which causes pain and stiffness.

Effects of temperature

Exercise is an effective way of increasing body temperature because when muscles are working they produce heat. When muscle tissue is warm, the muscle fibres contract more easily as the blood circulation is increased. Therefore the chemical reactions that naturally take place in the muscle cells are speeded up. When muscle tissue is cold, the opposite happens – the chemical reactions slow down and so contraction will be slower.

EFFECTS OF MASSAGE ON MUSCLES

- The blood supply to the muscle is increased during massage, bringing fresh oxygen and nutrients and removing waste products such as lactic acid, so massage can help to alleviate

---

Note

- **Myositis** is inflammation of a muscle.

- **Rupture** is a tearing or bursting of the fascia that surround the muscle.

- **Spasticity** refers to a spasm within one or more muscles. This is a problem associated with the nervous system.

- Overworking a muscle or a tendon can lead to a **strain**. There may be pain, swelling and stiffness.

muscle fatigue. The muscle is warmed because of the increased blood flow and, because warm muscles contract more efficiently than when cold, the likelihood of injury is reduced.

- Massage helps to relieve pain, stiffness and fatigue in muscles as the waste products are removed and normal functioning is quickly restored. The increased oxygen and nutrients aid tissue repair and recovery of the muscle.

- Massage can help the breakdown of fibrositic nodules, also termed **knots**, that develop within a muscle because of tension, injuries or poor posture. Knots are commonly found in the shoulder area.

- Massage helps to increase the tone of the muscles and delays wasting away of muscles through lack of use.

Task 4.1

Fill in the gaps in the following text.

- There are over ...6oo.... muscles in the body.
- The three types of muscle are .Cardiac........., ... and
....
- Skeletal muscles are an example of .... muscles.
- When a muscle contracts the thinner filaments, ..., slide in between the thicker filaments, called ....
- A .... nerve stimulates the muscle to contract.
- Muscle .... is the slight tension in which the muscles are continually held.
- When there is a low degree of muscle tone, the muscles are said to be
....
- When there is a high degree of muscle tone, the muscles are said to be
....
- Muscle fatigue occurs when there is insufficient .... and
....
- Stiffness and pain results when the waste products .... and
.... accumulate in the muscle.
- Injury to a muscle can cause complete or partial .... of the muscle fibres.
- Fibrositic nodules can develop as a result of ...., ... or
....

Look up the following terms in Chapter 3. They will help you to understand the actions of the muscles.

Term	Meaning
Flexion	....
	....
Extension	....
	....
Supination	....
	....
Pronation	....
	....
Lateral	....
	....
Medial	....
	....
Rotation	....
	....
Abduction	....
	....
Adduction	....
	....
Plantar	....
	....

Muscles of the head, face and neck

Task 4.3

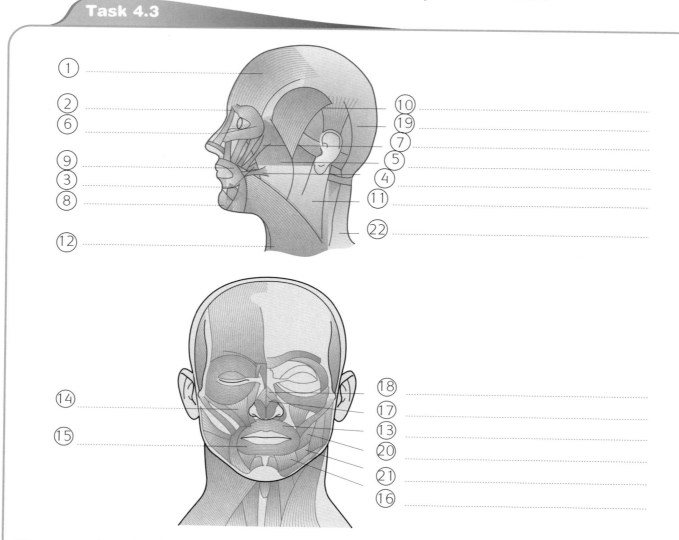

Figure 4.4 *Muscles of the face and neck*

Label the diagram in Figure 4.4 using the information in Table 4.1. Colour the muscles following this key:

Red – frontalis, risorius and sternocleidomastoid
Blue – corrugator, buccinator, occipitalis and splenius capitis
Yellow – orbicularis oculi, orbicularis oris and masseter
Orange – temporalis, platysma and levator anguli oris
Green – depressor anguli oris, nasalis and zygomaticus major
Brown – mentalis, levator labii superioris and triangularis
Purple – procerus, pterygoids and depressor labii inferioris.

Table 4.1 *Muscles of the head, face and neck*

Muscle	Position	Action
① Frontalis	Across the forehead	Draws scalp forward and raises eyebrows
② Corrugator	Between the eyebrows	Lowers eyebrows and wrinkles skin of forehead, as in frowning
③ Buccinator	In each cheek, to the side of the mouth	Compresses cheeks, as in whistling and blowing, and draws the corners of the mouth in, as in sucking
④ Risorius	Extends diagonally from either side of the mouth	Draws the corner of the mouth outwards, as in grinning
⑤ Masseter	The cheeks	The muscle of chewing: it closes the mouth and clenches the teeth
⑥ Orbicularis oculi	Around the eyes	Closes the eye
⑦ Zygomaticus major	Extends diagonally from the corners of the mouth	Lifts the corners of the mouth upwards and outwards, as in smiling or laughing
⑧ Mentalis	On the chin	Raises and protrudes lower lip, wrinkles skin on chin
⑨ Orbicularis oris	Surrounds the mouth	Closure and protrusion of the lips, changes shape of lips for speech
⑩ Temporalis	Extends from the temple region to the upper jaw bone	Raises the lower jaw and draws it backwards, as in chewing
⑪ Sterno-cleidomastoid	Runs from the top of the sternum to the clavicle and temporal bones	Both together bend head forward; one muscle only rotates the head and draws it towards the opposite shoulder
⑫ Platysma	Extends from the lower jaw to the chest and covers the front of the neck	Depresses lower jaw and draws lower lip outwards and draws up the skin of the chest
⑬ Levator anguli oris	On the cheek	Raises the corner of the mouth, as in smiling
⑭ Levator labii superioris	On the cheek	Lifts the upper lip, as in smiling
⑮ Depressor anguli oris	On the chin	Draws the corners of the mouth down, as in frowning
⑯ Depressor labii inferioris	On the chin	Lowers the bottom lip
⑰ Nasalis	Sides of the nose	Opens the nostrils, as when angry
⑱ Procerus	On the nasal bone	Causes the small horizontal lines between the eyebrows when angry
⑲ Occipitalis	At the back of the head	Draws the scalp backwards
⑳ Pterygoids (lateral and medial)	Outer part of the cheek	Moves the mandible from side to side, as in chewing
㉑ Triangularis	Chin	Lowers the corners of the mouth
㉒ Splenius capitis	Back of the neck	These muscles work together to move the head to an upright position

Origin and insertion

The **origin** of a muscle is the bone to which it is attached that does not move. The **insertion** is the bone to which the muscle is attached that does move. For example, the biceps of the upper arm has its point of origin at the shoulder, while the point of insertion is the radius of the lower arm. The insertion is the part farthest away from the spine. Muscles always move towards their origins.

Muscles in the body normally work in pairs to produce movement. During movement one muscle will contract while another relaxes:

- **prime mover** – the muscle or muscles that move and contract

- **antagonist** – the muscle or muscles that relax while the prime mover is contracting.

When we bend our forearm, the muscle at the front of the arm (the biceps) contracts, so it is called the prime mover. The muscle at the back of the arm (the triceps) relaxes, so it is called the antagonist (Figure 4.5).

> **Note**
>
> All of the muscles that are responsible for backward movements are to be found at the back of the body and all of the muscles concerned with forward bending are found at the front of the body. This will help you to remember the actions of the muscles.

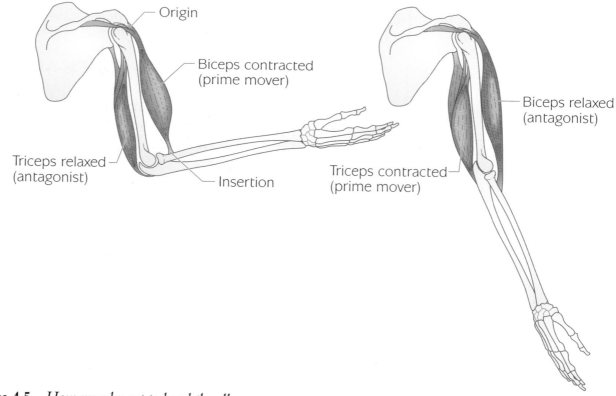

Figure 4.5 *How muscles act to bend the elbow*

Muscles of the shoulders

Deep muscles   **Superficial muscles**

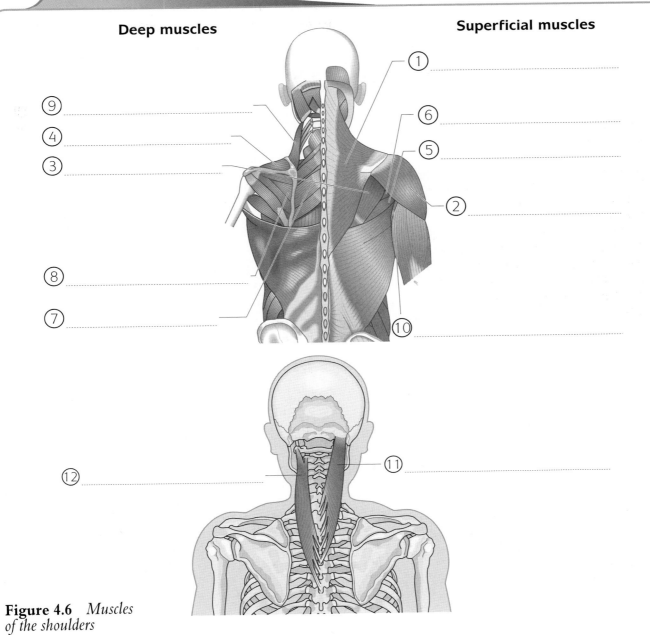

Figure 4.6 *Muscles of the shoulders*

Label the diagrams in Figure 4.6 using the information in Table 4.2. Use this key to colour the muscles:

Red – trapezius, coracobrachialis and supraspinatus
Yellow – deltoid, infraspinatus, splenius cervicis
Green – teres major and minor, rhomboids
Blue – subscapularis, levator scapulae and splenius capitis.

Table 4.2 *Muscles of the shoulders*

Muscle	Position	Origin	Insertion	Action
① Trapezius	Forms a large, kite-shaped muscle across the top of the back and neck	Occipital bone and vertebrae	Scapula and clavicle	Lifts the clavicle as in shrugging and also draws the head backwards
② Deltoid	A thick, triangular muscle that caps the shoulder	Clavicle and scapula	Humerus	Abducts the arm and draws it backwards and forwards
③ Infraspinatus	Deep muscle that covers the lower part of the scapula	Scapula	Humerus	Laterally rotates and adducts arm
④ Supraspinatus	Deep muscle that covers the upper part of the scapula	Scapula	Humerus	Helps deltoid muscle to abduct arm
⑤ Teres major	Deep muscle across back of shoulders	Scapula	Humerus	Helps medially rotate and adduct arm
⑥ Teres minor	Deep muscle across back of shoulders	Scapula	Humerus	Laterally rotates and adducts arm
⑦ Rhomboids	Between vertebral column and scapula	Thoracic vertebrae	Scapula	Rotate and adduct (pull) scapula towards spine
⑧ Subscapularis	Large, triangular muscle found beneath scapula	Scapula	Humerus	Medially rotates arm
⑨ Levator scapulae	At back and side of neck, on to scapula	Cervical vertebrae	Scapula	Lifts shoulder and scapula
⑩ Coracobrachialis	Upper medial part of arm	Scapula	Humerus	Flexes and adducts arm
⑪ Splenius capitis	Found under trapezius in the neck	Thoracic/cervical vertebrae	Occipital bone	Helps to hold neck and head in upright position and aids rotation of head
⑫ Splenius cervicis	Found beneath the splenius capitis	Thoracic vertebrae	Cervical vertebrae	Helps to hold up the head and neck and aids rotation of the head

Rotator cuff

The strength and stability of the shoulder joint are provided by the subscapularis, supraspinatus, infraspinatus and teres minor. These muscles join the scapula to the humerus. Their flat tendons join together to form a whole circle around the shoulder joint, like the cuff on a shirt sleeve.

Muscles of the posterior aspect of trunk

Task 4.5

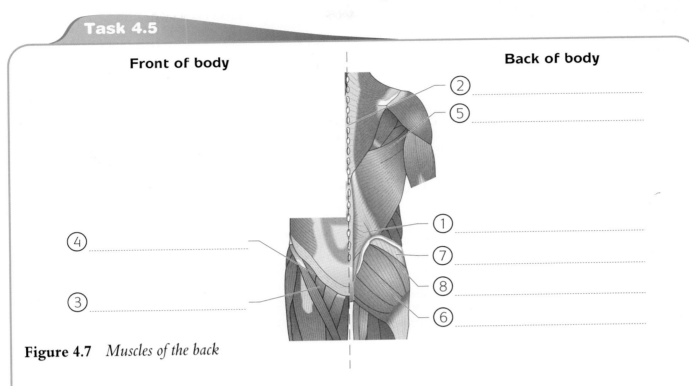

Figure 4.7 *Muscles of the back*

Label the diagram in Figure 4.7 using the information in Table 4.3. Use this key to colour the muscles:

Red – latissimus dorsi, gluteus maximus and psoas
Blue – iliacus and gluteus medius.

Table 4.3 *Muscles of the posterior aspect of the trunk*

Muscle	Position	Origin	Insertion	Action
① Quadratus lumborum	Deep muscle. Found medially on lower part of the back	Iliac crest	Ribs	Lateral flexion (side-bending) of lumbar vertebrae; assists diaphragm when breathing in
② Erector spinae	Three groups of deep muscles found on either side of vertebrae	Vertebrae, ribs, iliac crest	Cervical and lumbar vertebrae, ribs	Extends the spine and so helps to hold the body in an upright position
③ Psoas	In lumbar region of spine and across hip joint	Lumbar vertebrae/ sacrum	Femur	Flexes thigh and helps to laterally rotate thigh
④ Iliacus	Deep muscle of the pelvis that crosses hip joint	Ilium	Femur	Flexes thigh and helps to laterally rotate thigh
⑤ Latissimus dorsi (lah-tis'i-mus dor'se)	A large sheet of muscle down the back of the lower thorax and lumbar region	Vertebrae	Humerus	Draws the arm back and inwards towards the body; helps to pull body upwards when climbing
⑥ Gluteus maximus	Lower part of back forming buttocks	Ilium, sacrum, coccyx	Femur	Extends the hip and rotates thigh laterally; used in running and jumping
⑦ Gluteus medius	Lateral part of buttocks, deep to gluteus maximus	Ilium	Femur	Abducts and medially rotates the thigh, used in walking and running
⑧ Gluteus minimus	Lateral area of buttocks, beneath gluteus medius	Ilium	Femur	Abducts and rotates thigh, used in walking and running

Muscles of the upper limbs

Front of arm

Back of arm

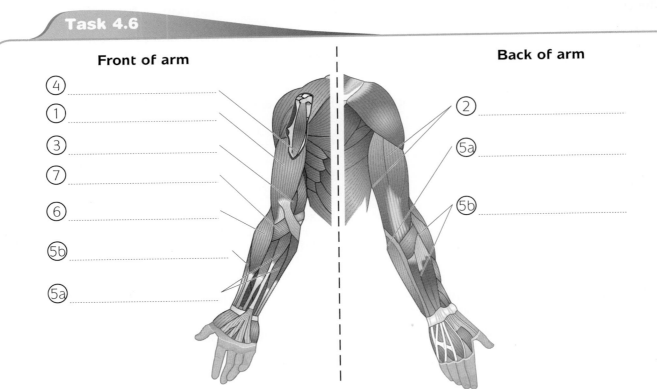

④ ....

① ....

③ ....

⑦ ....

⑥ ....

5b ....

5a ....

② ....

5a ....

5b ....

Figure 4.8 *Muscles of the upper limbs*

Label the diagram in Figure 4.8 using the information in Table 4.4. Use this key to colour the muscles:

Red – pronator teres, biceps
Yellow – flexors of forearm, triceps

Blue – extensors of the forearm
Orange – brachialis, brachioradialis.

Table 4.4 *Muscles of the upper limbs*

Muscle	Position	Origin	Insertion	Action
① Biceps brachii	Down anterior surface of the humerus	Scapula	Radius and flexor muscles in forearm	Flexes and supinates the forearm
② Triceps	Posterior surface of humerus	Humerus and scapula	Ulna	Extends the forearm
③ Brachialis (bra'ke-a-lis)	On the anterior aspect of humerus beneath the biceps	Humerus	Ulna	Flexes the forearm
④ Coracobrachialis	Upper arm	Scapula	Humerus	Flexes and adducts arm at shoulder joint
⑤a Flexors and ⑤b extensors of the forearm	Forearm	Flexors – humerus, radius and ulna Extensors – humerus	Carpals, metacarpals and phalanges	Flexors flex the wrist and extensors extend the wrist
⑥ Brachioradialis	On the same side as the radius bone of forearm	Humerus	Radius	Flexes, supinates and pronates forearm
⑦ Pronator teres	Anterior side of forearm, across elbow joint	Humerus and ulna	Radius	Pronates and flexes forearm

Muscles of the arms and hands

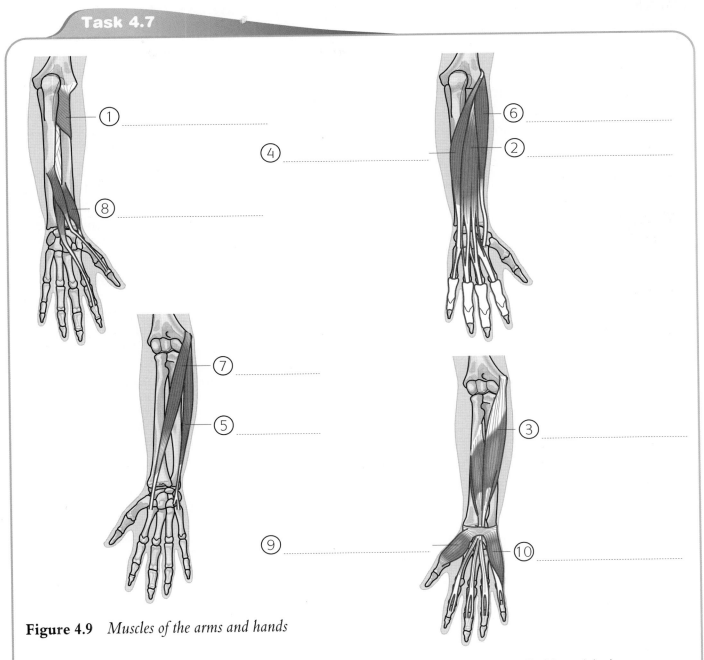

Figure 4.9 *Muscles of the arms and hands*

Label the diagrams in Figure 4.9 using the information in Table 4.5. Use this key to colour the muscles:

Red – supinator, muscles of thenar eminence
Yellow – extensor digitorum, extensor pollicis brevis
Blue – flexor digitorum superficialis, extensor carpi radialis
Orange – extensor carpi ulnaris, flexor carpi radialis
Green – flexor carpi ulnaris, muscles of hypothenar eminence.

Table 4.5 *Muscles of the arms and hands*

Muscle	Position	Origin	Insertion	Action
① Supinator	Forearm	Humerus	Radius	Supinates forearm
② Extensor digitorum	Forearm	Humerus	Phalanges	Extends phalanges
③ Flexor digitorum superficialis	Forearm	Humerus	Phalanges	Flexes phalanges
④ Extensor carpi ulnaris	Forearm	Humerus	5th metacarpal	Extends and adducts hand at wrist joint
⑤ Flexor carpi ulnaris	Forearm	Humerus	Carpals and 5th metacarpal	Flexes and adducts hand at wrist joint
⑥ Extensor carpi radialis	Forearm	Humerus	2nd metacarpal	Extends and abducts hand at wrist joint
⑦ Flexor carpi radialis	Forearm	Humerus	Metacarpals	Flexes and abducts hand at wrist joint
⑧ Extensor pollicis brevis	Forearm	Middle of radius	Phalanx of thumb	Extends phalanx of thumb at metacarpo-phalangeal joint
⑨ Muscles of thenar eminence	On the palm of the hand	Carpals and metacarpals	Phalanx of thumb	The four thenar muscles act on the thumb. Movements include adduction, abduction and flexion of the thumb
⑩ Muscles of hypothenar eminence	On the palm of the hand	Carpals	Phalanx of little finger and the metacarpal near to little finger	The three hypothenar muscles act on the little fingers. Movements include abduction and flexion of the little finger

Condition associated with the muscles of the arms and hand

Repetitive strain injury
Repetitive strain injury (RSI) includes conditions caused by the constant repetition of particular movements. It often affects typists and there may be pain or tingling when the fingers are moved. It is due to irritation of the flexor and extensor tendons in the wrist and hand. RSI can lead to another condition called **carpal tunnel syndrome**; this is due to pressure on the median nerve as it passes through a gap under a ligament at the front of the wrist.

Muscles of the anterior aspect of the trunk

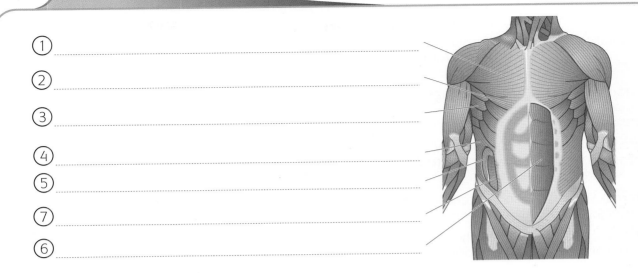

1 ....

2 ....

3 ....

4 ....

5 ....

7 ....

6 ....

Figure 4.10 *Muscles of the anterior trunk*

Label the diagram in Figure 4.10 using the information in Table 4.6. Use this key to colour the muscles:

Red – pectoralis major
Light blue – serratus anterior

Yellow – rectus abdominis
Orange – for the obliques.

Table 4.6 *Muscles of the anterior aspect of the trunk*

Muscle	Position	Origin	Insertion	Action
① Pectoralis major	Covers the upper part of the thorax	Sternum, ribs and clavicle	Humerus	Adducts and medially rotates the arm
② Pectoralis minor	Small muscle found beneath pectoralis major	Ribs	Scapula	Draws shoulder downwards and forwards
③ Serratus (ser-a'tis) anterior	Sides of ribcage below the armpits	Ribs	Scapula	Draws scapula forward as in pushing movements
④ External obliques	Found laterally from side of waist to anterior of abdomen	Ribs	Iliac crest and linea alba*	Twist trunk to opposite side
⑤ Internal obliques	Found laterally on anterior of abdomen	Iliac crest	Ribs and linea alba*	Twist trunk to opposite side
⑥ Rectus abdominis	Extends the whole length of the abdomen	Pubic bone	Sternum and lower ribs	Supports abdominal organs and flexes vertebral column (as in bending forwards)
⑦ Transversus abdominis (also known as trans versalis)	Found laterally on front of abdomen, beneath internal oblique muscle	Iliac crest, rib cage and vertebrae	The pubis, sternum and linea alba*	Supports abdominal organs and flexes vertebral column

*The linea alba is a tough, fibrous band that extends from the sternum to the pubis.

Muscles of the lower limbs

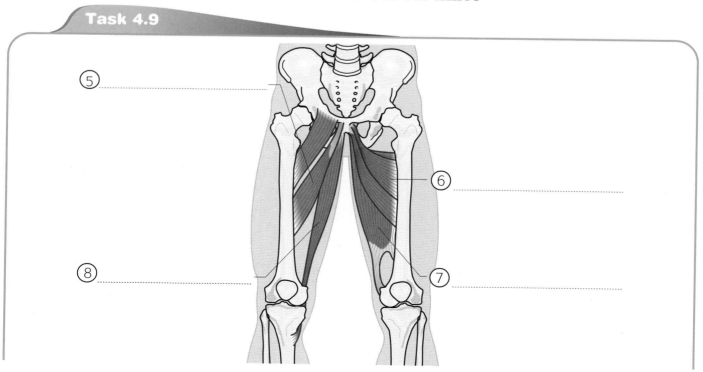

Task 4.9

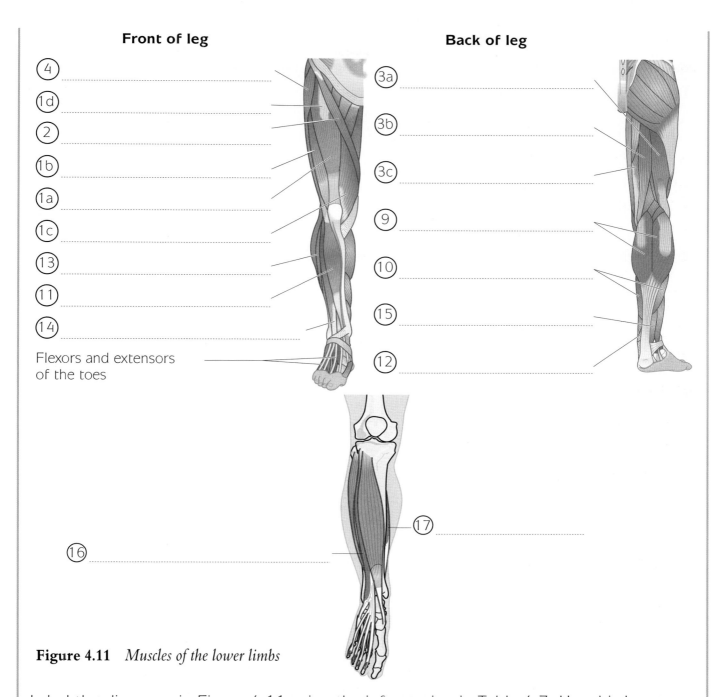

Front of leg

④
①d
②
①b
①a
①c
⑬
⑪
⑭

Flexors and extensors
of the toes

Back of leg

③a
③b
③c
⑨
⑩
⑮
⑫

⑯

⑰

Figure 4.11 *Muscles of the lower limbs*

Label the diagrams in Figure 4.11 using the information in Table 4.7. Use this key to colour the muscles:

Red – quadriceps and gastrocnemius
Light blue – hamstrings and tibialis anterior
Yellow – sartorius, tensor fasciae latae and soleus
Orange – adductors, peroneus longus
Green – tibialis posterior, flexor digitorum longus
Pink – extensor hallucis longus, extensor digitorum longus and flexor hallucis longus.

Table 4.7 *Muscles of the lower limbs*

Muscle	Position	Origin	Insertion	Action
① Quadriceps femoris	Group of four muscles located on the front of the thigh ⓐ rectus femoris ⓑ vastus lateralis ⓒ vastus medialis ⓓ vastus intermedius	Ilium and femur	Patella and tibia	Extends the leg and the rectus femoris, also flexes the thigh
② Sartorius	Crosses diagonally on anterior aspect of thigh	Ilium	Tibia	Flexes knee and hip, and rotates the thigh laterally
③ Hamstrings	Group of three muscles situated on the back of the thigh ⓐ biceps femoris ⓑ semitendinosus ⓒ semimembranosus	Ischium	Tibia	Flex the knee and extend the hip
④ Tensor fasciae latae	Along lateral side of thigh	Ilium	Tibia	Abducts and flexes the thigh
⑤ Adductor longus	Medial side of thigh	Pubis and ischium	Femur	Adducts and flexes thigh at hip, medially rotates thigh
⑥ Adductor brevis	Medial side of thigh	Pubis	Femur	Adducts and fexes thigh at hip, medially rotates thigh
⑦ Adductor magnus	Medial side of thigh	Pubis and ischium	Femur	Adducts thigh, anterior part flexes thigh and posterior part extends thigh
⑧ Gracilis (adductor muscle)	Medial side of thigh	Pubic bone	Tibia	Adducts the thigh and flexes the leg at the knee joint
⑨ Gastrocnemius	Back of lower leg	Femur	Calcaneum in the foot via the Achilles tendon	Plantarflexes the foot (draws the foot downwards)
⑩ Soleus	At back of lower leg, deep to gastrocnemius	Tibia and fibula	Calcaneum via the Achilles tendon	Plantarflexes foot
⑪ Tibialis anterior	Down the shin bone	Tibia	Tarsal and metatarsal bones	Dorsiflexes the foot (draws the foot upwards)
⑫ Tibialis posterior	Deepest muscle on back of lower leg	Tibia and fibula	Metatarsals, navicular, cuneiforms and cuboid	Plantarflexes and inverts foot (turns foot inwards)

⑬ Peroneus longus	Down the outside of lower leg	Fibula	First metatarsal and cuneiform bone	Plantarflexes and inverts foot (turns foot outwards); supports the transverse and lateral longitudinal arches of the feet
⑭ Extensor hallucis longus	Down front of lower leg	Fibula	Phalanx of big toe	Extends the big toe
⑮ Flexor hallucis longus	Outer side and towards the back of lower leg	Fibula	Phalanx of big toe	Flexes the big toe, inverts and plantarflexes foot; also supports medial longitudinal arch of foot
⑯ Extensor digitorum longus	Lateral to tibialis anterior muscle	Tibia, fibula	Phalanges	Dorsiflexes foot
⑰ Flexor digitorum longus	Medial to tibialis anterior muscle	Tibia	Phalanges	Plantar flexes foot

Task 4.10

Copy Tables 4.1 to 4.6. Mix up the names, origins and insertions, positions and actions and try to match them back together.

Note

The tendons of the muscles are held firmly in place by the superior extensor retinaculum (transverse ligament of the ankle) and the inferior extensor retinaculum (cruciate ligament of the ankle).

POSTURE

A good posture means that the body is aligned and balanced, so that the work carried out by muscles to maintain it is kept to a minimum. It will ensure that muscles and joints are working efficiently so that the body remains free from muscular tension, strains, stiffness and pain. A poor posture means that the body is out of balance so that certain muscles have to contract strongly to maintain it. Over a period of time these muscles will tighten and shorten, while others will stretch and weaken. Three main postural faults are lordosis, kyphosis and scoliosis (Figure 4.12).

Lordosis

Lordosis is a condition that shows itself as an inward exaggeration of the lumbar region of the spine. The client will appear to have a hollow back and there will be protrusion of the abdomen and buttocks. Gymnasts often adopt this posture.

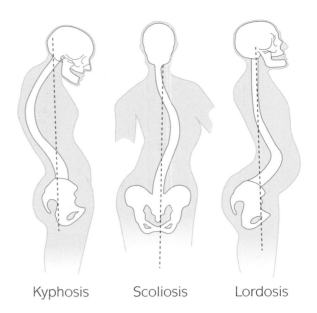

Figure 4.12 *Postural faults*

Kyphosis   Scoliosis   Lordosis

- **Weak muscles** The hamstrings, gluteus maximus, rectus abdominis, internal and external oblique muscles are stretched and lengthened.
- **Tight muscles** The muscles of the lumbar region are shortened and the gluteal muscles weakened.

Kyphosis

Kyphosis is a condition where there is an exaggeration of the thoracic curve of the spine. The client will have rounded shoulders and the chin pokes forwards. Adopting a poor posture often causes kyphosis.

- **Weak muscles** The upper back muscles are weakened and overstretched.
- **Tight muscles** The pectoral muscles are tightened and shortened.

Scoliosis

A feature of scoliosis is a lateral curvature of the spine, which may be C- or S-shaped. It can result in the level of the shoulders and pelvic girdle being slightly uneven. An individual may be born with this condition or the continual carrying of heavy bags on one particular shoulder over a period of time can cause it. The muscles that are shortened are found on the inside of the curve and the muscles that are overstretched will be found on the outside of the curve. Shortened and tight muscles can be relaxed and stretched with massage which can help to correct posture faults.

The circulatory systems 5

The cardiovascular system consists of the heart, blood and blood vessels. The function of the heart is to act as a pump to move the blood around the body. The blood carries oxygen and nutrients and is transported in the body by blood vessels.

BLOOD AND ITS FUNCTIONS

Blood plasma

Plasma is the liquid part of the blood and mainly consists of water. Many substances can travel in the blood plasma, including blood cells, hormones, nutrients and the waste products produced by cells. Plasma proteins are also found in the blood.

Plasma proteins include albumin, globulin and fibrinogen, which are all made in the liver. Clotting factors are also plasma proteins and, along with fibrinogen, help to clot the blood to prevent bleeding.

Functions of the blood

The blood has several functions. It:

- **distributes** oxygen, nutrients and hormones to the cells of the body. Heat is also transported around the body from the muscles and liver, which helps regulate the body temperature
- **removes** carbon dioxide and waste from the cells
- **attacks** harmful organisms such as bacteria. The white blood cells protect the body against disease
- **clots** the blood to prevent excessive loss of blood if an injury occurs to the body.

Blood cells

Red blood cells

Red blood cells (**erythrocytes**) are button-shaped cells that are made in the bone marrow and live for about three months.

> **Note**
>
> To help you remember the functions of the blood think of **D-R-A-C**-ula:
>
> **D** – distributes
> **R** – removes
> **A** – attacks
> **C** – clots.

Fact!

There are approximately five million red blood cells in a drop of blood.

There are approximately five million of these cells in a drop of blood. Red blood cells contain the pigment **haemoglobin**. The oxygen picked up from the lungs combines with the haemoglobin.

The function of red blood cells is to carry oxygen around the body and deliver it to the cells. The cells use the oxygen and nutrients and produce carbon dioxide. Carbon dioxide can be carried away by the red blood cells and taken back to the lungs to be breathed out.

Fact!

Lack of iron leads to a condition called anaemia.

Haemoglobin is rich in iron and needs a constant supply of it. Iron comes from the food we eat and also from old or damaged red blood cells that have been destroyed by the liver. Lack of iron leads to a condition called **anaemia**; symptoms include tiredness, dizziness and shortness of breath.

Lymphocyte
(white blood cell)

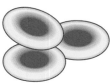
Erythrocytes
(red blood cells)

Thrombocytes
(platelets)

Figure 5.1 *Blood cells*

White blood cells

White blood cells (**leucocytes**) contain a nucleus and are larger than red blood cells. There are up to 10,000 in a drop of blood. Most types of white blood cell can change their shape so they are able to squeeze through small spaces. Therefore, white blood cells are able to reach almost anywhere in the body. The function of white blood cells is to protect us from disease. Leukaemia is a cancer caused by the overproduction of white blood cells.

Fact!

Leukaemia is a cancer of the blood and is caused by the overproduction of white blood cells.

Leucocytes are made up of granulocytes and agranulocytes:

- About 75 per cent of white blood cells are made in the bone marrow; these cells are called **granulocytes** because they have tiny granules in their cytoplasm. Most granulocytes are **phagocytes** – this means that they are able to engulf and digest (eat) bacteria and any other harmful matter.

- **Agranulocytes** do not have granules in their cytoplasm. These white cells make up the remaining 25 per cent and are mostly produced in the lymphatic system. Lymphocytes and monocytes are types of agranulocyte:

Note

An **autoimmune disease** is one in which antibodies, produced by the immune system, attack the body's own tissues. Examples include arthritis, psoriasis and multiple sclerosis.

– The job of **lymphocytes** is to produce antibodies. Antibodies are chemicals made by the body in response to bacteria and any other harmful matter. They have the function of destroying the harmful matter so that it is no longer a threat to the body.

– **Monocytes** also destroy harmful matter, e.g. bacteria, by engulfing and digesting it, like most of the granulocytes. These cells gather around wounds and kill invading bacteria to prevent them from entering the body.

Platelets

Platelets (**thrombocytes**) are tiny fragments of cells, which are smaller than white and red blood cells. They are produced in the bone marrow and live for up to two weeks. There are about 200,000 in a drop of blood. Platelets are involved with the clotting process of the blood following an injury to the body. Their function is to help to prevent loss of blood from damaged blood vessels by forming a plug.

Blood clotting

A blood clot is formed at the site of an injury to the body and prevents the loss of further blood. If this process did not occur we would bleed to death. In haemophiliacs the blood clots very slowly, so a great deal of blood may be lost from even small cuts. Clotting factors can be injected so that haemophiliacs can lead a normal life.

Stages of blood clotting

1 A wound to the skin stimulates the platelets to release an enzyme called **thromboplastin** (Figure 5.2 A). (An enzyme is a protein that speeds up chemical reactions.)

2 Thromboplastin converts a protein found in the blood plasma called **prothombin** into another enzyme known as **thrombin**. Vitamin K and calcium are also needed for this process (Figure 5.2 B).

3 Thrombin will act on a soluble protein, also found in the blood plasma, called **fibrinogen**. Thrombin converts fibrinogen into an insoluble substance called **fibrin**. Fibrin consists of fibrous strands, which form a net (Figure 5.2 C). The blood cells become trapped in the net and so a blood clot is formed.

4 The clot dries out to form a scab, which is a natural plaster to protect the skin underneath (Figure 5.2 D).

Figure 5.2 *Stages of blood clotting*

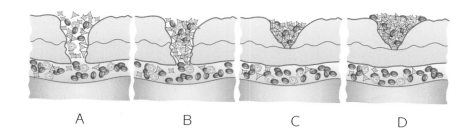

A   B   C   D

THE HEART

The heart is situated between the lungs in the thoracic cavity (chest region), lying slightly to the left of the body. It is roughly the size of its owner's closed fist and is an organ made up mainly of cardiac muscle.

The heart consists of four chambers: the **right atrium**, **left atrium**, **right ventricle** and **left ventricle**. The upper chambers are together called the **atria** and the lower chambers of the heart are called the **ventricles**.

The heart also contains valves to prevent the blood from flowing backwards. The right side of the heart is separated from the left side by a muscular wall called the **septum** (Figure 5.3). Blood

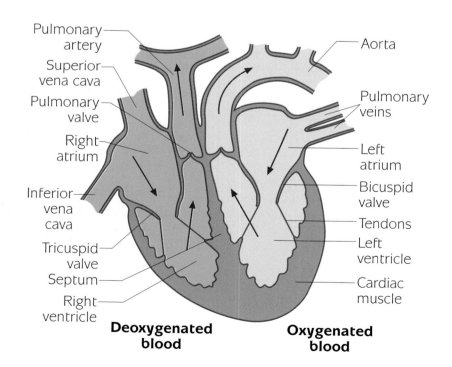

Figure 5.3 *A simplified cross-section showing the structure of the heart and how blood passes through it (see also Figure 1.3)*

that passes through the right side of the heart is known as **deoxygenated blood** because it carries very little oxygen. The blood that passes through the left side of the heart is rich in oxygen so is called **oxygenated blood**. Blood vessels that transport blood away from the heart are called **arteries**, while blood is brought to the heart in **veins**.

The heart wall consists of three layers:

- The **endocardium** is the inner layer of the heart wall.

- The **myocardium** is the middle layer of the heart and contains the cardiac muscle that contracts to pump the blood.

- The **pericardium** is the outer layer of the heart.

PULMONARY CIRCULATION

The pulmonary circulation is the circulation of blood between the heart and the lungs.

- Deoxygenated blood travels through veins called the **inferior vena cava** and **superior vena cava** into the right atrium.

- Blood flows from the right atrium through a valve and into the right ventricle.

- From the right ventricle the blood passes through another valve and travels into the **pulmonary arteries**.

- From the pulmonary arteries the blood is carried to the lungs. An exchange of gases occurs in the lungs. The blood gets rid of the carbon dioxide, which is breathed out and a fresh supply of oxygen is picked up from the lungs. The blood now becomes oxygenated.

- The oxygenated blood is then returned to the left atrium of the heart by the **pulmonary veins**.

GENERAL (SYSTEMIC) CIRCULATION

The general circulation is the circulation of blood from the left side of the heart to the rest of the body's tissues.

- The oxygenated blood passes from the left atrium through a valve and into the left ventricle.

- The blood leaves the left ventricle of the heart and passes into a large blood vessel (artery) called the **aorta**. The blood, which also transports nutrients, is then carried around the body to supply oxygen and nutrients to all the cells. Carbon dioxide is picked up from the tissues and the blood now contains little oxygen, so it becomes deoxygenated again.

- The deoxygenated blood is eventually returned to the right atrium of the heart by the superior vena cava and inferior vena cava.

Task 5.1

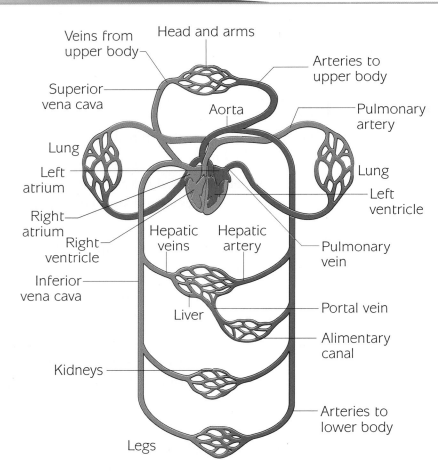

Figure 5.4 *The pulmonary circulation and the systemic circulation*

Read the sections on the pulmonary and general circulation and draw arrows on the diagram in Figure 5.4 to show how blood circulates around the body. Use red arrows for the oxygenated blood and blue for the deoxygenated blood.

Note

- Coronary heart disease is caused by the blockage of the arteries that carry blood to the heart muscle. This is a condition called **atherosclerosis**. The arteries become furred up with a fatty substance called **cholesterol**, which causes a decrease of blood flow to the heart.

- **Arteriosclerosis** is hardening of the arteries. The term **atherosclerosis** is generally used instead.

Blood is transported around the body in a series of pipes called **blood vessels** (Figure 5.5). These blood vessels are called arteries, arterioles, capillaries, venules and veins, and form an intricate network within the body.

Arteries

Arteries have thick, elastic, muscular walls because the blood within them is carried under high pressure because of the pumping action of the heart. Arteries carry blood **away** from the heart. All arteries carry **oxygenated** blood, with the exception of the pulmonary arteries which carry deoxygenated blood from the heart to the lungs. Arteries are generally deep-seated except where they cross a pulse spot, such as the radial artery in the wrist and carotid artery in the neck where a pulse can be felt. As arteries get further from the heart they branch off and become smaller. The oxygenated blood eventually reaches very small arteries called **arterioles**.

Capillaries

Arterioles are connected to the capillaries. Capillaries are the smallest vessels, about a hundredth of a millimetre thick. Unlike arteries and veins, the walls of the capillaries are thin enough to allow certain substances to pass through them – this is known as **capillary exchange**. Oxygen and nutrients are delivered to the cells of the body and carbon dioxide and waste products are removed.

The capillaries connect with larger vessels called **venules**. Now that oxygen has been removed from the blood and carbon dioxide has been picked up, by the time the blood reaches the venules it has become deoxygenated (Figure 5.7).

Veins

Blood flows through the venules until it reaches larger vessels called veins. The veins carry blood, called venous blood, towards the heart. Their walls are thinner and less elastic than arteries. Veins carry deoxygenated blood, with the exception of the pulmonary veins which carry oxygenated blood from the lungs to the heart. Veins are nearer the surface of the body than the arteries. Unlike the other blood vessels, veins contain valves which prevent the blood from flowing backwards.

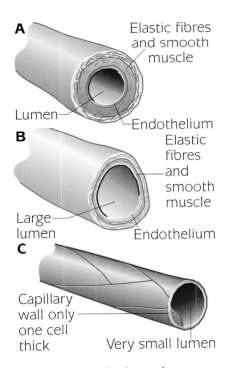

A Elastic fibres and smooth muscle

Lumen

Endothelium

B Elastic fibres and smooth muscle

Large lumen

Endothelium

C Capillary wall only one cell thick

Very small lumen

Figure 5.5 *Blood vessels: A artery, B vein, C capillary*

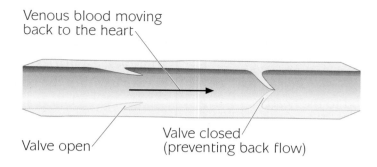

Venous blood moving back to the heart

Valve open

Valve closed (preventing back flow)

Figure 5.6 *Valves in the veins*

Unlike arteries, the veins carry blood at low pressure because they are not helped by the pumping action of the heart. Blood in the veins is moved through the body by the squeezing action of the voluntary muscles, such as during walking, and the involuntary muscles, such as the movement of breathing. Therefore, exercise and massage are particularly useful to help the venous flow.

Task 5.2

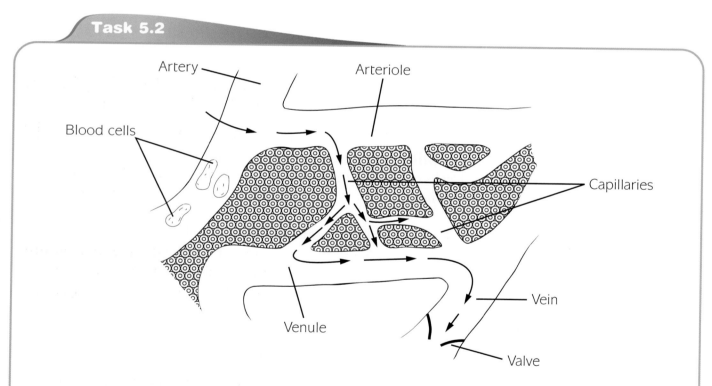

Artery

Arteriole

Blood cells

Capillaries

Venule

Vein

Valve

Figure 5.7 *How blood passes from arteries through capillaries to veins*

In the diagram in Figure 5.7, colour the artery and arteriole red, the veins and venule blue, and the capillaries yellow.

Fill in the table showing the differences between arteries and veins.

	Arteries	Veins
Thickness of walls	....	....
Pressure of blood	....	....
Do they have valves?	....	....
Blood carried oxygenated/deoxygenated?	....	....
Blood to heart/away from heart?	....	....
How blood is moved along vessels	....	....
Deep-seated or near surface of body?	....	....

Blood supply of the head and neck

To the head and neck – arteries

The blood to the head arrives via the **carotid arteries**. There are two main carotid arteries, one either side of the neck:

① the **internal carotid artery**, which supplies oxygenated blood to the brain

② the **external carotid artery**, which carries blood to the more superficial structures of the head, i.e. muscle, skin and bone.

Important arteries of the head and neck include the ③ **common carotid**, the ④ **occipital**, the ⑤ **superficial temporal**, the ⑥ **maxillary**, the ⑦ **facial**, the ⑧ **lingual** and the ⑨ **thyroid** arteries.

From the head and neck – veins

Important veins of the head and neck include the ① **middle temporal**, the ② **superficial temporal**, the ③ **maxillary**, the ④ **anterior facial**, the ⑤ **common facial**, the ⑥ **internal jugular**, the ⑦ **external jugular** and the ⑧ **occipital** veins.

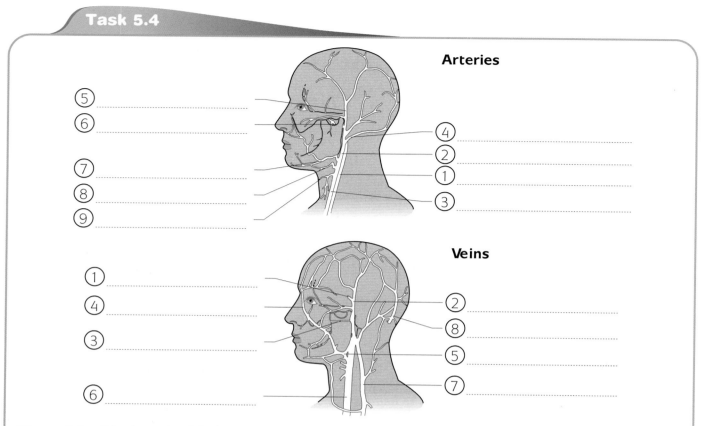

Figure 5.8 *Blood vessels of the head and neck*

Label the diagrams in Figure 5.8 using the information on page 99. Colour the arteries in red and the veins in blue.

Main blood vessels of the body

The ① **aorta** is the largest artery of the body; its diameter is about the size of a ten pence piece. This artery subdivides to become smaller arteries and supplies blood to the whole body.

The ② **inferior vena cava** is the largest vein in the body, about 3.5 cm in diameter. The ③ **superior vena cava** has a diameter about the size of a ten pence piece.

Other important blood vessels include: ④ **pulmonary artery**, ⑤ **pulmonary vein**, ⑥ **hepatic portal vein**, ⑦ **hepatic artery**, ⑧ **hepatic vein**, ⑨ **renal artery**, ⑩ **renal vein**.

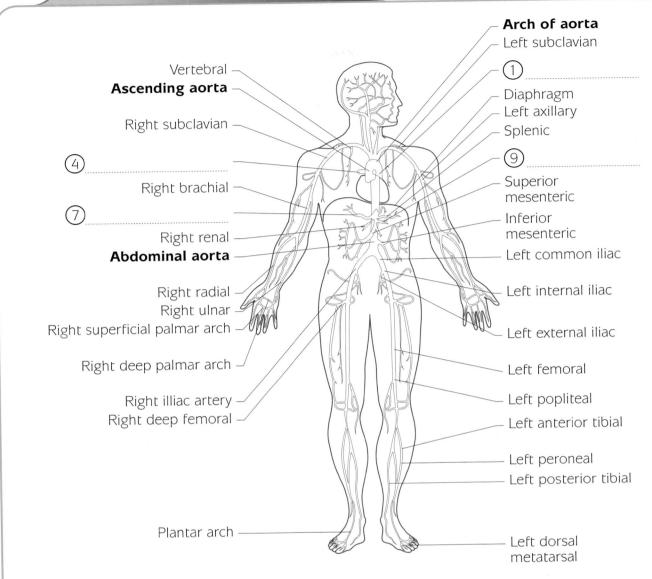

Vertebral
Ascending aorta
Right subclavian
④ ....
Right brachial
⑦ ....
Right renal
Abdominal aorta
Right radial
Right ulnar
Right superficial palmar arch
Right deep palmar arch
Right iliac artery
Right deep femoral
Plantar arch

Arch of aorta
Left subclavian
① ....
Diaphragm
Left axillary
Splenic
⑨ ....
Superior mesenteric
Inferior mesenteric
Left common iliac
Left internal iliac
Left external iliac
Left femoral
Left popliteal
Left anterior tibial
Left peroneal
Left posterior tibial
Left dorsal metatarsal

Figure 5.9 *Arteries of the body*

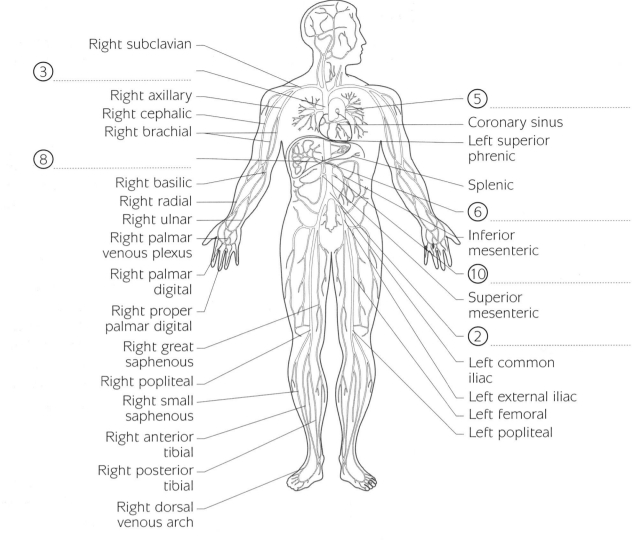

Figure 5.10 *Veins of the body*

Label the diagrams in Figures 5.9 and 5.10 using the information on page 100. Colour the arteries in red and the veins in blue.

Conditions associated with the systemic circulation

Varicose veins

If valves in the veins stop functioning properly a condition called varicose veins can result. The veins become permanently dilated (widened) as the valves can no longer prevent blood from flowing backwards down them. The blood pools in the veins and causes them to swell and bulge. Varicose veins commonly occur in the veins near the surface of the leg. They can also occur in the anus and here they are called haemorrhoids or piles. The causes of varicose veins include hereditary factors, ageing, obesity, pregnancy and jobs that involve long periods of standing. The affected veins must not be touched during treatment.

Thrombosis

A thrombosis is a clot of blood that is stationary within an artery or vein. It is dangerous as it may constrict or cut off the flow of blood. If massage is carried out there is a risk that the clot may be moved or broken up and taken to the heart, lungs or brain, which could prove fatal.

Embolism

This is a blockage of an artery with a clot of material that is contained within the bloodstream. A piece broken away from a thrombosis can be the cause. It circulates in the bloodstream until it becomes wedged somewhere in a blood vessel and blocks the flow of blood. Such a blockage may be extremely harmful. Do not treat clients with thrombosis or embolism, and if they have a history of these conditions it may be wise to check with their doctor before treatment.

Phlebitis

This is an inflammation of the walls of veins caused by tiny blood clots. There is redness, tenderness and swelling along the affected veins. No treatment should be given to anyone suffering with this condition.

HIV/AIDS

HIV (human immunodeficiency virus) is the cause of AIDS. HIV destroys or damages many of helper T-lymphocytes, which play an important part in the defence against other viruses, bacteria and fungi. In fully developed AIDS, immunity is lost. Therefore the body becomes susceptible to illness.

Hepatitis A, B, C

Hepatitis is inflammation of the liver. This is mainly caused as a result of a viral infection but can also be caused by alcohol and drugs. There are many types of virus responsible for hepatitis.

- **Hepatitis A** virus is a common infection in many parts of the world. It can be caught through eating or drinking contaminated food or water.

- **Hepatitis B** is very infectious and the virus can be spread through unprotected sex, sharing contaminated needles and using non-sterilised equipment for tattooing and body piercing.

- **Hepatitis C** can be caught through contaminated needles, non-sterilised equipment for tattooing etc. and unprotected sex.

If a person continues to be infected over a number of years, they could develop chronic hepatitis, liver cirrhosis or liver cancer.

The symptoms of Hepatitis A, B, C are similar and include flu-like illness, nausea, vomiting, diarrhoea and jaundice (yellow skin and whites of eyes).

HOW THE CIRCULATION WORKS

The cardiac cycle

The technical name for the contraction of the heart is **systole**. Systole begins as a wave of muscle contraction running down and across the atria from left to right, forcing blood into each of the ventricles. A fraction of a second later, the wave reaches the ventricles and they too contract, forcing blood into the aorta and pulmonary arteries.

After the heart has contracted, the atria and ventricles relax, known as **diastole**. The atria again fill with blood and the cardiac cycle starts again. One systole and one diastole form what is known as a **cardiac cycle**. It is one complete heartbeat and lasts for 0.8 seconds.

Blood pressure

When blood reaches the capillaries, it is vital that oxygen and nutrients pass out of the blood and into the cells. It is the pressure of blood that forces fluid out through the capillary walls. The fluid contains oxygen and nutrients that pass into the cell by diffusion. Therefore, it is important for the body to maintain the correct level of blood pressure.

With each heartbeat, the atria and ventricles contract (systole). As a chamber of the heart contracts, the blood pressure inside it will increase. Blood pressure measures the force with which the heart pumps blood around the body. It is the force of pressure the blood exerts against the walls of the arteries. Blood pressure can be

> **Note**
>
> To help you remember diastole, think of **DR** (doctor) – **D** is for diastole and **R** for relaxation, as the atria and ventricles relax during diastole.

likened to the pressure in a hosepipe which increases and decreases as the tap is turned on and off. The blood pressure varies during a complete heartbeat.

A doctor uses a sphygmomanometer to measure this blood pressure. Two phases of blood pressure are measured:

- **systolic pressure** – the force exerted by blood on the walls of the arteries during the contraction of the ventricles, which shows the highest pressure the heart can produce. It is the first number in a blood pressure reading and also the first sound heard as the large heart valves close

- **diastolic pressure** – the measure of the pressure on the walls of the arteries during relaxation of the ventricles. It is the second number in a blood pressure reading and is the lowest blood pressure measured in the large arteries. At this time the smaller heart valves close, producing the second, quieter heartbeat.

A normal blood pressure will measure around 120 mmHg systolic and 80 mmHg diastolic, or 120/80.

Blood pressure is used as an indicator of the health of the blood vessels and heart. Damaged blood vessels that are less elastic or have a partial blockage will show a raised blood pressure and a weak heart will show low blood pressure. People who exercise regularly often have slightly lower-than-normal blood pressure. Exercise helps to strengthen the heart, so it has to do less work to pump the same amount of blood.

High/low blood pressure

High blood pressure (**hypertension**) is when the blood pressure is consistently above normal. It can lead to strokes and heart attacks as the heart has to work harder to force blood through the system. High blood pressure can be caused by smoking, obesity, lack of exercise, eating too much salt, stress, too much alcohol, the contraceptive pill, pregnancy and hereditary factors.

Low blood pressure (**hypotension**) is when the blood pressure is below normal for a substantial time. Blood pressure must be sufficient to pump blood to the brain when the body is in the upright position. If it is not then the person will feel faint. Some people with low blood pressure may feel faint when sitting up suddenly from the lying position. The causes of low blood pressure include Addison's disease, loss of blood and heart conditions.

Fact!

People who exercise regularly often have slightly lower-than-normal blood pressure.

Note

A high intake of salt in the diet causes water to be retained in the body. This may result in an increased amount of blood in the body, and so lead to raised blood pressure, as the heart has to work harder to pump the extra blood around the body.

Pulse

The pulse can be felt in arteries that lie close to the surface of the body, such as the radial artery in the wrist and the carotid artery in the neck. The number of pulse beats per minute represents the heart rate. The pumping action of the left ventricle in the heart is strong so it can be felt as a pulse in arteries. The average pulse of an adult at rest is between 60 and 80 beats per minute.

Factors affecting the pulse rate

- **Exercise** Any form of exercise will cause the pulse rate to increase. During strenuous exercise, the pulse rate can double.

- **Emotion** The pulse rate can increase at times of stress, excitement, fear, anger and any other strong emotional states.

- **Age** Children have a higher pulse rate than adults.

- **Gender** The pulse rate in males is higher than in females.

- **Drugs** Certain drugs can influence the pulse rate.

Tachycardia means a fast resting heart or pulse rate that beats over 100 times per minute. If a person has tachycardia while at rest, too much coffee or tea, certain drugs, anxiety or fever may be the cause. Sometimes it can be a symptom of coronary heart disease.

Bradycardia means a slow resting heart or pulse rate of less than 60 beats per minute. Athletes who compete in endurance sports normally have bradycardia.

Effects of adrenalin on the heart

The hormone adrenalin is released from the adrenal glands which sit on top of each kidney. Adrenalin is released in response to stress, fear, exercise and excitement. It causes the heart rate to speed up and the coronary blood vessels to dilate, increasing the blood supply to the heart muscle. The increase in blood pressure means that a greater volume of blood is pumped with each beat, allowing more blood to reach vital organs and muscles.

Control of heart rate by nerves

The cardiac muscle of the heart has the ability to contract without the need of a nerve supply from the brain. If removed from the body, it can still continue to contract as long as it is provided with oxygen. The heart has a built-in pacemaker, so it will naturally beat at between 60 and 100 beats per minute. However, nerves are able to control the rate at which the heart beats. Nerves called

Fact!

The heart has a built-in pacemaker, so it will naturally beat at between 60 and 100 beats per minute.

sympathetic nerves can cause the heart rate to speed up and **parasympathetic nerves** can cause the heart rate to slow down.

Whether at rest or undertaking exercise, the sympathetic and parasympathetic nerves ensure that the heart rate can be adjusted to meet demands. When at rest, the parasympathetic nerve will cause the heart rate to beat at about 75 beats per minute, which is the average heart rate for a person.

Control of blood pressure by nerves

Nerves can control the diameter of the blood vessels. If the blood pressure is too low, the sympathetic nerves of the autonomic nervous system cause the blood vessels to contract. Contraction of these vessels leads to a decrease in the diameter of the vessels. This causes the pressure of blood inside the vessels to increase so that the blood pressure can return to normal. If the blood pressure is too high, the muscles in the walls of the blood vessels will relax so that the diameter of the vessels increases. This will cause the blood pressure to be lowered and so return to normal.

Blood shunting

The body contains about 60,000 miles of blood vessels and there is not enough blood to fill them all at any one time. There are certain points along some of the blood vessels where the small arteries have direct connection with veins. Vessels called **shunt vessels** provide this short cut and allow blood from the artery to enter the vein, so bypassing the capillaries (Figure 5.11).

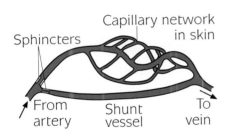

Figure 5.11 *Blood shunting*

Note

Massage increases the circulation to the skin and muscles, so it is not advised to have this treatment after eating a big meal.

Blood shunting can occur in the body while exercising and after eating a heavy meal. During exercise, the body becomes hot and so blood is brought to the skin. This ensures that heat is lost from the body so it may cool down. After eating a heavy meal, blood is directed to the intestines in the abdomen to help with digestion of the food. This means there is less supply of blood in other areas of the body and is why we can feel tired after eating a heavy meal.

Blood groups

A person's blood can be classified as belonging to a particular blood group. During a blood transfusion, if the blood groups of the donor and patient (recipient) are not compatible, the red blood cells clump together, known as **agglutination**. This results in a blockage of the blood vessels, and therefore can be fatal.

Table 5.1 *The compatibility of blood groups*

Type	May give to	May receive from
O	Any blood group	O
A	A and AB	O and A
B	B and AB	O and B
AB	AB	Any blood group

Most people have blood which belongs to one of four groups: A, B, AB and O (Table 5.1).

◦ In the UK, O is the most common blood group.

◦ Type O is the **universal donor** because it can be given to a patient with either type A, B or AB blood. If a patient has blood group type O they can only receive type O.

◦ Type AB is called the **universal recipient** because a patient with this type can receive blood from all blood groups. A donor with type AB blood can only give to people with type AB blood.

EFFECTS OF MASSAGE ON THE CIRCULATORY SYSTEM

Massage causes the blood vessels to be compressed, forcing blood forward. As pressure is released, the blood vessels return to their normal size and blood rushes in to fill the space created. Reddening of the skin, called **erythema**, results. Fresh, oxygenated blood and nutrients are brought to the area and so will nourish the tissues and help with tissue repair. Waste products (metabolic waste) are removed and carried away by the veins. A build-up of waste products can cause pain and stiffness and so massage can help to relieve these symptoms.

Massage movements such as effleurage (stroking) will help to return the blood in the veins back to the heart (venous return). This is why strokes are performed in the direction of the venous flow.

THE LYMPHATIC SYSTEM

Have you noticed that certain glands swell up when you are ill, such as the glands in the neck, which inflame during a throat infection? The glands you can feel are lymph nodes. Lymph nodes, lymph, lymph vessels and lymphatic ducts all make up the lymphatic system, which is closely related to blood circulation.

How is lymph derived?

Blood does not flow into the tissues but remains inside the blood vessels. However, plasma from the blood is able to seep through the capillary walls and enter the spaces between the tissues. This fluid provides the cells with nutrients and oxygen. It has now become tissue fluid, also known as interstitial fluid. More fluid passes out of the blood capillaries than is returned to the blood. The excess tissue fluid passes into the lymphatic capillaries and now becomes **lymph**. Lymph is similar to blood plasma but contains more white blood cells (Figure 5.12).

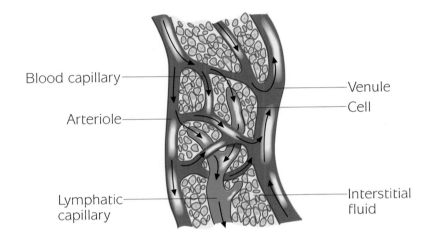

Figure 5.12 *The relationship between blood and lymph*

The functions of the lymphatic system

- **Helps to fight infection** The lymphatic system is an important part of the body's immune system. It produces specialised white blood cells called **lymphocytes**, which recognise harmful substances and destroy them.

- **Distributes fluid in the body** Lymphatic vessels drain approximately 3 litres of excess tissue fluid daily from tissue spaces.

- **Transport of fats** Carbohydrates and protein are passed from the small intestine directly into the bloodstream. However, fats are passed from the small intestine into lymphatic vessels called **lacteals** before eventually passing into the bloodstream.

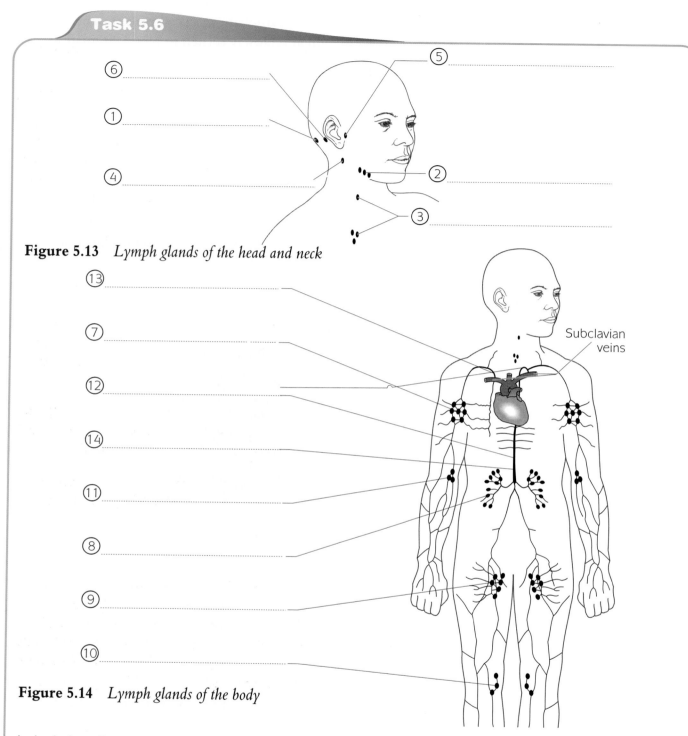

Figure 5.13 *Lymph glands of the head and neck*

Subclavian veins

Figure 5.14 *Lymph glands of the body*

Label the diagrams in Figures 5.13 and 5.14 using the information on pages 111 and 112. Use this key to colour the diagrams:

Yellow – the lymph glands and lymphatic vessels
Green – the thoracic and right lymphatic duct
Red – the subclavian veins and heart.

Lymph nodes

There are approximately 600 bean-shaped lymph nodes scattered throughout the body. They lie mainly in groups around the groin, breast, armpits and round the major blood vessels of the abdomen and chest.

Lymph is a watery, colourless fluid that passes through the lymph nodes. Lymph nodes filter out harmful substances from the lymph, such as bacteria, which could cause an infection in the body. They contain specialised white blood cells called monocytes and lymphocytes:

- **Monocytes** destroy harmful substances by ingesting (eating) them.

- **Lymphocytes** produce antibodies that stop the growth of bacteria and prevent their harmful action. During an infection there are more bacteria and so the lymph nodes produce more lymphocytes to destroy them. This causes the lymph nodes to enlarge and is a sign that the glands are working to fight the infection.

Important groups of lymph nodes in the head are: the ① **occipital**, ② **submandibular**, ③ **deep cervical** and ④ **superficial cervical glands**, ⑤ **anterior auricular** and ⑥ **posterior auricular**.

Important groups of lymph nodes in the rest of the body include the ⑦ **axillary**, ⑧ **abdominal**, ⑨ **inguinal**, ⑩ **popliteal** and ⑪ **supratrochlear** nodes.

Structure of lymph nodes

Lymph nodes have a fibrous outer capsule containing lymphoid tissue. Lymph enters the node through the **afferent lymphatic vessels** and leaves the node via the **efferent lymphatic vessels**. As many as five afferent lymph vessels may enter a node while only one or two efferent vessels carry lymph away from it. **Trabeculae** divide the node into sections, provide support and enable blood vessels to enter into the node (Figure 5.15).

Lymph vessels

Lymph travels around the body in one direction only, towards the heart. It is carried in vessels that begin as **lymphatic capillaries**. Lymph capillaries are blind-ended tubes, situated between cells, and are found throughout the body. The walls of lymphatic capillaries are structured in such a way that tissue fluid can pass into them but not out of them.

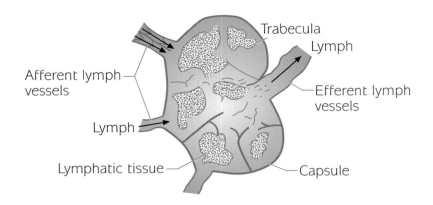

Figure 5.15 *Structure of a lymph gland*

Lymphatic capillaries join up and become wider tubes, known as **lymphatic vessels**. The lymph vessels generally run parallel to the veins. These vessels are similar to veins as they contain valves, although they generally have thinner walls. The lymph flows around the body through these lymph vessels and passes through a number of lymph nodes to be filtered. Eventually the lymph will be passed into lymphatic ducts.

Lymphatic ducts

The lymphatic ducts are known as the ⑫ **thoracic duct** and ⑬ **right lymphatic duct**. The thoracic duct is approximately 40 cm long. Lymph vessels from the lower body join up to form a large lymph vessel called the ⑭ **cisterna chyli**, which leads to the thoracic duct. The cisterna chyli is situated in front of the first two lumbar vertebrae. The thoracic duct is the main collecting duct of the lymphatic system. It receives lymph from the left side of the head, neck and chest, the upper limbs and the whole body beneath the ribs. The thoracic duct drains the lymph directly into the left subclavian vein, so that it is returned back to the blood circulation (Figure 5.16).

The right lymphatic duct is about 1.25 cm long and drains lymph from the upper right hand side of the body. The lymph passes into the right subclavian vein, where it joins the venous blood to become part of the blood circulation once again.

The lymphatic system does not have a pump like the heart, but like veins relies on the movement of the body and the contraction of the skeletal muscles. The squeezing action of the muscles forces the lymph along its vessels. Involuntary actions such as breathing and the heartbeat also help the movement of lymph through the vessels.

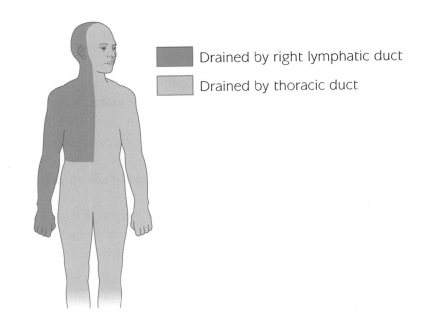

Drained by right lymphatic duct

Drained by thoracic duct

Figure 5.16 *Lymph drainage*

Tonsils, adenoids and Peyer's patches are made from lymphatic tissue. **Tonsils** are found in the throat and **adenoids** are found at the back of the nose. They help to destroy bacteria and other harmful matter as air is taken into the body. **Peyer's patches** are found in the small intestine and also help to destroy harmful substances to help prevent infection.

Task 5.7

Decide the order of sequence of the events described below and place the correct letter in each box.

A   Tissue fluid passes into lymphatic capillary.
B   Plasma now becomes tissue fluid.
C   Tissue fluid now becomes lymph.
D   Tissue fluid provides the cells with nutrients and oxygen.
E   Plasma in the blood seeps through the capillary wall.

1	2	3	4	5

The spleen

The spleen consists of lymphatic tissue and is part of the lymphatic system. It is oval in shape and weighs approximately 200 g. The spleen is situated in the left side of the abdomen, beneath the diaphragm and behind the stomach. The normal adult spleen is about the size of a large apple.

Functions of the spleen

- The spleen acts as a reservoir for blood. If blood is needed elsewhere in the body, perhaps because of a haemorrhage, it can be diverted.

- Lymphocytes are produced here, so the spleen is an important part of the immune system. If the spleen has to be removed, resistance to disease may be slightly lowered.

- The spleen has a good blood supply. Old, worn-out red blood cells are filtered from the blood and destroyed after their 120-day life.

The spleen can be easily damaged by trauma. If this happens a haemorrhage can occur so the damaged spleen has to be removed quickly. The body can still survive without it.

Conditions associated with the lymphatic system

Hodgkin's disease

This is cancer of the lymph nodes, which become enlarged all over the body. The cause is unknown, but cancer-causing viruses are thought to be involved.

Oedema (fluid retention)

Fluid retention is a common problem in which there is an accumulation of excess fluid in the body tissues. Depending on the cause, it can either be localised (affecting only a certain part of the body) or generalised (affecting the whole body). Fluid retention causes swelling, which is commonly seen around the ankles. It can be differentiated from other types of swelling by the fact that slight pressure will leave a dent in the skin which takes a few seconds to return to normal. It often occurs in women just before a period and also in the last three months of pregnancy. It can also be a symptom of high blood pressure or injury, and a side-effect of certain drugs.

The respiratory and olfactory systems

6

THE RESPIRATORY SYSTEM

Every living cell in the body needs oxygen. We obtain the oxygen we require from the air that we breathe. **Inspiration** is the movement of air into the lungs and **expiration** is the movement of air out of the lungs. The respiratory system is concerned with the exchange of gases between the lungs and the blood and consists of a number of organs.

Task 6.1

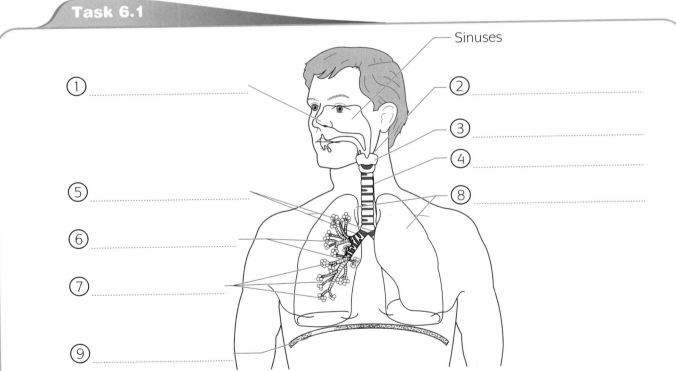

Figure 6.1 *Respiratory organs*

Label the diagram in Figure 6.1 matching the numbers to the numbered terms in the following text. Use this key to colour the respiratory organs:

Red – nose, sinuses, pharynx, larynx, trachea, bronchi and bronchioles
Yellow – alveoli and diaphragm
Brown – the lungs
Blue – diaphragm.

① Nose

Air is breathed in through the nose and becomes moistened and warmed. Coarse hairs filter out large dust particles. In the nasal cavity there are tiny, hair-like structures called **cilia**. A sticky substance called **mucus** is produced by cells called **goblet cells** and helps to trap dust particles. The cilia transport the mucus with the trapped dust particles towards the pharynx (throat) where they are swallowed and destroyed by acid in the stomach.

The **sinuses** are hollow spaces within the bones of the skull that open into the nasal cavity. These spaces are filled with air and are lined with a mucous membrane. Infection or allergy causes these membranes to become swollen, leading to excessive mucus production and a watery discharge.

② Pharynx (throat)

The pharynx is a tube and acts as an air and food passage. It allows air to enter the larynx and food to enter the food pipe. The larynx is anterior to the food pipe. The **tonsils** are found at the back of the pharynx. They are made up of lymphoid tissue and their job is to filter bacteria in the same way as lymph nodes.

The throat is connected to an area of the ear, known as the **middle ear**, by the **eustachian** (u-stay-she-an) **tube**. Bacteria in the throat can pass through the eustachian tube causing a painful middle-ear infection.

③ Larynx

Note

The closing of the epiglottis while swallowing ensures (most of the time) that the food will enter the food pipe rather than the windpipe, otherwise choking will result.

The larynx is the voice box and is a short passageway linking the pharynx to the trachea. It consists of cartilages the largest of which forms the Adam's apple. During swallowing, the pharynx and larynx rise. A piece of flap-like cartilage called the **epiglottis** acts as a lid to cover the opening of the larynx.

④ Trachea (windpipe)

The trachea or windpipe is a tube that acts as a passageway for air. It is held open by up to 20 C-shaped rings of cartilage, which give the trachea some rigidity to ensure that there is no obstruction of airflow. The trachea extends into the thorax (chest cavity) and branches off to form the bronchi.

Note

During exercise, the action of the sympathetic nervous system increases and the adrenal glands produce adrenalin, which causes the muscles within the bronchi to relax so the airways are dilated. This results in a quicker supply of air to the alveoli.

Fact!

Each lung contains approximately 150 million alveoli.

⑤ Bronchi

The bronchi are two tubes, each individually known as a **bronchus**, which carry air into the lungs. Like the trachea, they contain cartilage rings that keep the tubes fairly rigid to ensure adequate airflow.

The trachea and bronchi contain cilia and cells that produce mucus. The mucus and cilia trap dust and other harmful substances. The cilia waft to and fro and carry the mucus and dust towards the throat, where it is swallowed and then dealt with by acid in the stomach.

⑥ Bronchioles

The bronchi divide into branches called bronchioles. The bronchioles become progressively smaller until they join on to the alveoli.

⑦ Alveoli

Alveoli are round, sac-like structures and their shape ensures a large surface area for exchange of gases. The alveoli have very thin walls and each alveolus is surrounded by a network of capillaries: this ensures that an efficient exchange of oxygen and carbon dioxide can take place.

⑧ Lungs

The lungs are large organs situated at either side of the thoracic cavity and separated by the heart. They are each enclosed in a **pleural membrane** which consists of two layers: the **visceral** (vis-er-al) **pleura** and **parietal pleura**. Between these layers is a space called the **pleural cavity**, containing fluid. The fluid allows the membranes to slide over each other during breathing, preventing friction.

⑨ Diaphragm

The diaphragm is a large, dome-shaped muscle found directly under the lungs. It separates the thoracic cavity from the abdominal cavity. The diaphragm plays a major role in breathing and helps to ensure that the thoracic cavity is airtight.

Match the terms in the bubbles with the correct description in the list:

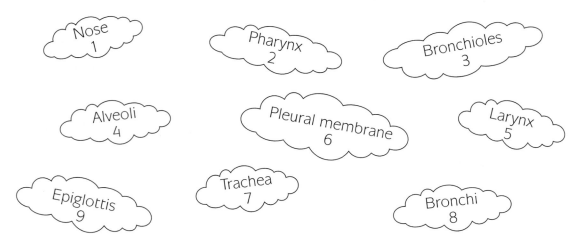

Nose 1

Pharynx 2

Bronchioles 3

Alveoli 4

Pleural membrane 6

Larynx 5

Epiglottis 9

Trachea 7

Bronchi 8

- The throat ....
- Round sac-like structures ....
- Prevents food from entering trachea during swallowing ....
- Membrane surrounding a lung ....
- Two tubes that enter each lung ....
- Small tubes that branch out in the lungs ....
- Moistens and warms the air breathed in ....
- Contains the voice box ....
- Windpipe ....

Gas exchange in the lungs

Air is breathed into the lungs where oxygen diffuses through the walls of the alveoli and into the blood. It is picked up by the red blood cells and taken around the body to provide oxygen for the body's cells. The cells produce carbon dioxide, which has to be removed from the body. The carbon dioxide diffuses from the cells into the surrounding capillaries. When it reaches the capillaries surrounding the alveoli, it passes through the walls of the alveoli and is breathed out. The deoxygenated blood becomes oxygenated once again. This is a process that is continually happening and is essential for life (Figure 6.2).

Fact!

Essential oils used in aromatherapy are also able to pass into the bloodstream through the respiratory system.

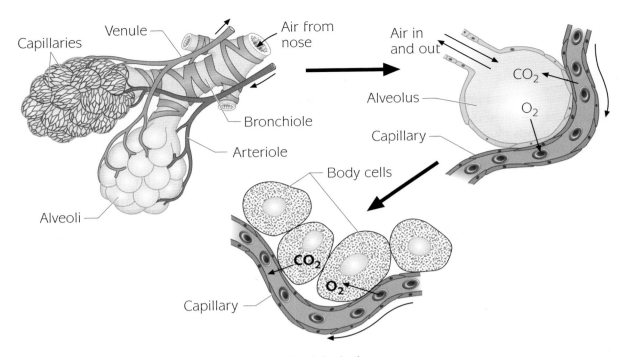

Figure 6.2   *Gas exchange in the lungs and in the cells of the body*

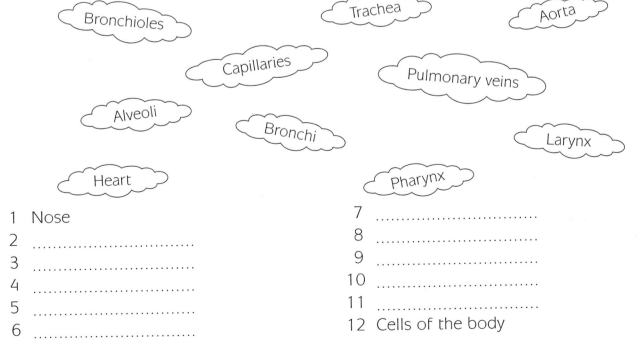

Task 6.3

Air firstly travels through the nose and finally the oxygen reaches the cells of the body. What is the pathway of oxygen through the body? Write the names of the organs from the bubbles on the correct line of the list below. You may need to refer back to Chapter 5.

Bronchioles   Trachea   Aorta

Capillaries   Pulmonary veins

Alveoli   Bronchi   Larynx

Heart   Pharynx

1 Nose
2 ....
3 ....
4 ....
5 ....
6 ....

7 ....
8 ....
9 ....
10 ....
11 ....
12 Cells of the body

The mechanism of breathing

During inspiration, the external intercostal muscles found between the ribs contract, moving the ribs up and out. The diaphragm muscle also contracts and so the dome shape is flattened. This increases the space in the lungs and causes air to be automatically drawn into them.

During expiration, the external intercostal muscles relax and the ribs return to their resting position. The diaphragm relaxes, returning to its original dome shape. This causes the space in the lungs to get smaller, forcing air out of them (Figure 6.3).

Note

This process can be likened to having your hands glued to a balloon (which represents the lung attached to the chest wall) and pulling it wider to increase the space inside.

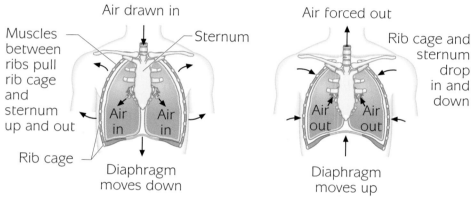

Figure 6.3
The mechanism of breathing

Role of brain in respiration

Breathing is controlled by the **medulla oblongata** in the brain. Messages are sent from the brain, through phrenic nerves to the diaphragm, and by the intercostal nerves to the external intercostal muscles, and cause these muscles to contract. This causes us to breathe in. When the messages stop, relaxation of the muscles occurs, and so expiration takes place.

Chemical control

When exercising, you require more oxygen, therefore the body produces more carbon dioxide as the cells produce it as a by-product. The body needs to get rid of this carbon dioxide, and does so by increasing the breathing rate. **Chemoreceptors** are found in the medulla oblongata and in the walls of the aorta and carotid arteries. They are sensitive to carbon dioxide levels in the blood. When stimulated, they send messages to the respiratory centres in the brain, which leads to an increase in the breathing rate.

The effect of smoking on the respiratory system

Cigarette smoking has the following effects on the respiratory system:

- It coats the inside of the lungs with tar so they become inefficient.

- It covers the cilia in tar preventing them from getting rid of bacteria from the lungs.

- It leads to diseases such as emphysema and bronchitis.

- It causes lung cancer. Most patients with lung cancer have been smokers.

Conditions associated with the respiratory system

Rhinitis

Rhinitis is an inflammation of, and discharge from, the mucous membranes in the nose. The swelling of the membrane blocks the free flow of air though the nose. Rhinitis is a symptom of the common cold, hayfever and sinus problems.

Hayfever

Caused by an allergy to certain pollens, the hayfever season begins in early spring and lasts until late autumn. Symptoms include a runny nose, sneezing and itchy eyes.

Sinusitis

Sinusitis is an inflammation of the membrane lining the sinuses. Infections such as a cold can result in sinusitis, in which there is a painful, throbbing feeling in the cheeks and behind the nose and eyes.

Asthma

This is a condition in which the muscles of the bronchi go into a state of spasm so that the bronchi are narrowed causing difficulty in breathing. The cause may be due to an allergy, infection, exercise or stress.

Bronchitis

Bronchitis is inflammation of the bronchi. Symptoms include a cough, shortness of breath and wheezing. Cigarette smoke is the main cause of chronic bronchitis.

Emphysema

This is a disorder in which the walls of the alveoli are destroyed thus producing abnormally large air spaces which remain filled with air during breathing out so breathing becomes very difficult. Common causes include cigarette smoking and air pollution.

Pleurisy

Pleurisy is the inflammation of the pleura and is usually caused by a viral or bacterial infection, and can be the result of pneumonia.

Pneumonia

This is inflammation of the lungs. It can be caused by a viral or bacterial infection.

Tuberculosis

Tuberculosis (TB) is a bacterial infection which can affect the lungs or other parts of the body such as the bones, skin and heart. Symptoms include fever, persistent cough, chest pain and tiredness.

THE OLFACTORY SYSTEM

Fact!

A professional perfumier can distinguish 100,000 different odours.

The olfactory system provides us with the sense of smell also known as **olfaction**. The brain is able to distinguish about 20,000 different scents with the help of the nervous system. Millions of olfactory receptors in the nose transmit messages in the form of nerve impulses to the brain.

How is smell perceived?

Substances such as essential oils (oils used in aromatherapy) give off ① **smelly gas particles**. These particles are drawn into the nose as we inhale and dissolve into the upper part of the moist mucous membrane of the nasal cavity.

The ② **mucus** surrounds small hairs called ③ **cilia** that stick out from the bottom of ④ **olfactory cells**. The gas particles reach the cilia and stimulate nerve impulses to travel along the ⑤ **axon of the nerve cell**, through bones in the skull and to the ⑥ **olfactory bulb**, of which there are two.

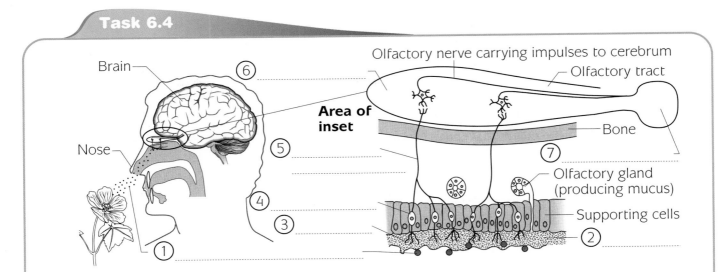

Task 6.4

Figure 6.4 *The olfactory system*

Label the diagram in Figure 6.4 matching the numbers to the numbered terms in the text on pages 122–3. Use this key to colour the diagram:

Green – mucus

Blue – olfactory cell, cilia and axon

Yellow – olfactory bulb

Red – the limbic system.

Nerves from the olfactory bulb then carry nerve impulses to the brain, many of which are part of the ⑦ **limbic system.** The limbic system is involved with emotions such as pain, anger, pleasure, affection and memory. This is why smells can evoke different emotional responses and can bring back a flood of memories.

Adaption

We can become adapted to a smell. If we spray perfume, we will soon stop noticing its smell because the olfactory receptors, of which there are millions, will stop being stimulated until a new smell comes along.

Note

The olfactory receptor consists of the olfactory cell, cilia and axon.

Decide the order of sequence of the events described below and place the correct letter in each box.

A   Smell is perceived in the olfactory area of the brain.
B   Particles of substance are in the air.
C   Olfactory cells connect directly with the brain.
D   Particles stimulate olfactory cells.
E   Particles dissolve in mucous layer in nasal cavities.

1	2	3	4	5

The nervous system

The nervous and endocrine systems work together to maintain a stable internal environment (**homeostasis**) within the body. The nervous system consists of the brain, spinal cord, nerves and sense organs. It controls all the bodily systems and provides the most rapid means of communication in the body.

Millions of nerve impulses (messages) are continually reaching the brain from receptors in, for instance, the skin, and just as many leave the brain and stimulate muscles to move and organs to carry out their work. In the body the messages are in the form of electrical impulses which pass from neurone (nerve cell) to neurone. There are billions of **neurones** within the body and their function is to transmit nerve impulses.

NEURONES

The cell body contains a nucleus and branches of nerve fibres called **dendrites** (Figure 7.1). Dendrites carry the impulses towards the cell body and on to the **axon**. Therefore impulses always move in one direction only. Each neurone has only one axon, but this can be anything from 1 mm long to over 1 m long.

The axon is covered in a fatty **myelin sheath**. The myelin sheath insulates the neurone to prevent loss of the electrical impulses, and also increases the speed at which the impulse is conducted. Some (**unmyelinated**) nerve cells do not have a myelin sheath. Nerve cells with a sheath are able to transmit impulses 200 times faster than unmyelinated ones. The myelin sheath consists of a series of **Schwann cells** arranged along the length of the axon. The outer layer of the Schwann cell membrane is sometimes called the **neurilemma**. Gaps occur in the myelin sheath and are called **nodes of Ranvier**, which help to ensure the impulses (messages) are carried quickly from neurone to neurone.

Note

The nervous system can be likened to a telephone network with messages continually being passed through wires.

Fact!

There are billions of neurones within the body and their function is to transmit nerve impulses.

Fact!

Each neurone has only one axon, but this can be anything from 1 mm long to over 1 m long.

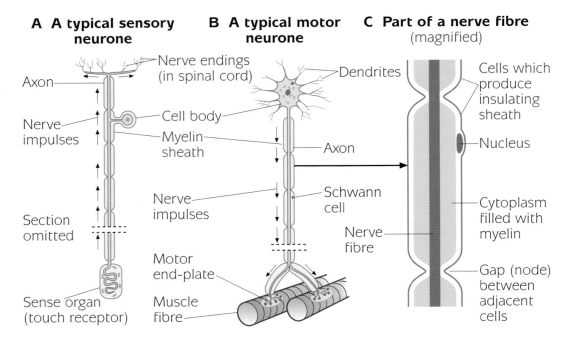

Figure 7.1 *Structure of a nerve cell*

Fact!

The fastest nerve signals can travel at 250 mph.

HOW IMPULSES ARE TRANSMITTED

Neurones transmit nerve impulses to other neurones or organs such as muscles. When two neurones meet there is a gap between them called a **synapse** (Figure 7.2). The nerve impulse is transferred to the next neurone by the release of chemicals, which diffuse across the synapse. The chemicals then set off a new electrical signal in the next neurone.

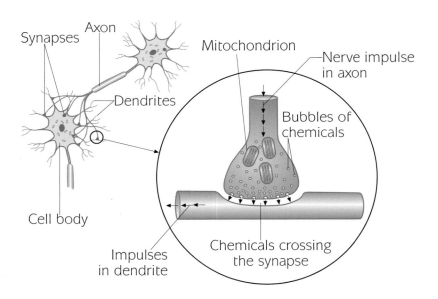

Figure 7.2 *Structure of a synapse*

Match the terms in the bubbles with the correct description in the list:

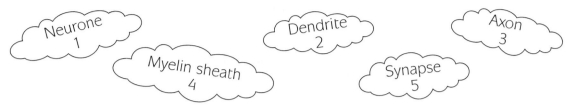

Neurone
1

Dendrite
2

Axon
3

Myelin sheath
4

Synapse
5

- Gap in between two neurones ....
- Fatty insulating material ....
- Branch from the cell body ....
- Carries impulses away from cell body ....
- Nerve cell ....

NERVES

The axons from a large number of neurones are arranged in bundles and form **nerves** (Figure 7.3). Nerves are rather like electrical wires surrounded by cable. A **ganglion** (plural: ganglia) is a group of nerve cell bodies which are located outside the brain and spinal cord.

Unlike other cells, neurones cannot divide and reproduce themselves. If neurones are destroyed they cannot be replaced although they can be repaired if damaged.

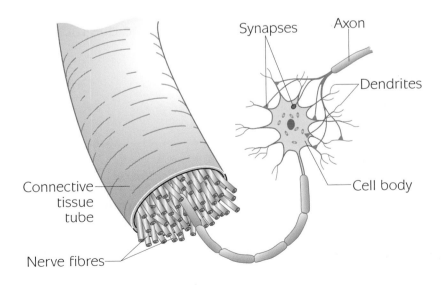

Figure 7.3 *Structure of a nerve*

DIVISIONS OF THE NERVOUS SYSTEM

The nervous system can be divided into the central, peripheral and autonomic nervous systems.

Central nervous system (CNS)

The central nervous system consists of the brain and spinal cord. The brain is the most important part of the system and contains 100 billion neurones. The brain receives and stores messages as well as transmitting them to all parts of the body to stimulate organs to do their work.

Task 7.2

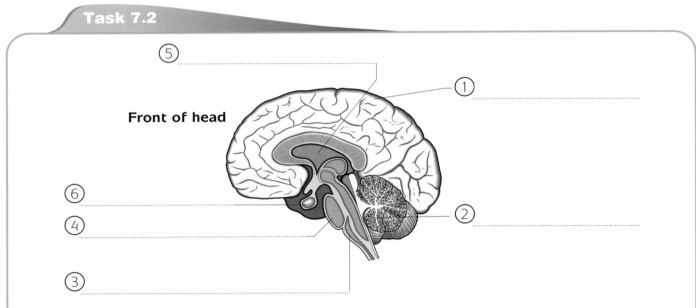

Front of head

Figure 7.4 *Structures in the brain*

Label the diagram in Figure 7.4 matching the numbers to the numbered terms in the following text. Use this key to colour the diagram:

Yellow – cerebrum
Pink – cerebellum
Orange – medulla oblongata

Blue – pons varolii
Green – thalamus
Red – hypothalamus.

① *Cerebrum*

The cerebrum is the largest portion of the brain. It is a dome-shaped area of nervous tissue split into two halves:

♦ the **left hemisphere**, which controls the right side of the body. In most people the left hemisphere is more important for language, numerical and scientific skills

Note

The brain stem is made up of three parts: the **medulla oblongata**, the **pons varolii** and the **mid-brain**. The mid-brain is found between the cerebrum and cerebellum.

Fact!

The medulla oblongata is responsible for vomiting, which basically involves squeezing the stomach between the diaphragm and abdominal muscles.

♦ the **right hemisphere**, which controls the left side of body. The right side is the creative side and is important for musical and artistic ability.

The **grey matter** on the surface of the brain is made up of nerve cell bodies and is where the main functions of the cerebrum are carried out. These include all conscious activities such as touch, taste, smell, hearing, vision and all voluntary muscular movement. The cerebrum also controls the powers of reasoning, learning, emotion and memory.

The **white matter** of the brain and spinal cord consists of nerve fibres (axons) in white myelinated sheaths.

② *Cerebellum*

The cerebellum deals with movement. It helps to control our balance and posture. It maintains muscle tone and co-ordinates muscles during activities such as walking and running. It is also responsible for learning skills such as playing the piano or riding a bike.

③ *Medulla oblongata*

The medulla oblongata is a mass of grey matter. It regulates the heart and breathing rates, constriction and dilation of the blood vessels, body temperature and the reflex actions of sneezing, coughing, vomiting and swallowing.

④ *Pons varolii*

The pons varolii forms a bridge (*pons* is Latin for 'bridge') that transmits messages between the spinal cord, cerebellum and cerebrum.

⑤ *Thalamus*

The thalamus co-ordinates impulses from sense organs such as the skin, eyes, nose and taste buds before they reach the cerebrum.

⑥ *Hypothalamus*

The hypothalamus controls the activities of the autonomic nervous system (see page 138) and an endocrine gland called the **pituitary gland**. The hypothalamus is one of the main regulators of homeostasis, helping to maintain a constant internal environment in the body.

The functions of the hypothalamus include the control of many body functions:

- Through the autonomic nervous system it controls blood pressure, heart rate, contraction of the bladder and the movement of food through the alimentary canal.

- With the help of the kidneys it controls the salt and water balance of the body.

- It controls hunger and thirst to ensure sufficient intake of water and nutrients into the body.

- It controls the body temperature by acting like a thermostat. If the temperature of the blood flowing through the hypothalamus is above normal, the hypothalamus instructs the autonomic nervous system to promote heat loss by means of, for example, sweating and vasodilation. If the blood temperature is below normal, the hypothalamus causes the body to shiver to produce heat.

- Together with the limbic system it controls the feelings associated with aggression, pain, pleasure and sexual arousal.

- It helps to maintain waking and sleeping patterns.

Neuroglia

The spaces between neurones are filled with cells called **neuroglia**, which support the neurones, provide nutrients and help them to conduct nerve impulses. Two types of neuroglia are:

- **Astrocytes** Many of these star-shaped cells are found in the brain lying next to blood vessels. Astrocytes only allow certain substances to pass from the blood into the brain. This is known as the **blood–brain barrier** and protects the brain cells from most harmful substances. Certain substances, such as oxygen, glucose and also carbon dioxide, alcohol and nicotine, pass quickly across this barrier into the brain. It is thought that essential oils can also pass through the blood–brain barrier.

- **Oligodendrocytes** These cells form a supporting network around the nerve cells of the central nervous system. They also produce the myelin sheath for these nerve cells.

Spinal cord

The spinal cord is continuous with the medulla oblongata, extending downwards through the vertebral column and ending level with the lumbar vertebrae. It contains about 100 million

Note

Meningitis is inflammation of the meninges.

neurones. As in the brain, coverings called **meninges**, made up of three connective tissue layers, protect it. The layers are called **pia**, **arachnoid** and **dura mater**.

The spinal cord contains white and grey matter. Grey matter appears as a butterfly shape in the middle of the spinal cord and is surrounded by white matter.

The **cerebrospinal fluid** (CSF) is similar to blood plasma in composition. It protects the brain and spinal cord by acting as a cushion and shock absorber between the brain and the cranial bones. It also keeps the brain and spinal cord moist and provides nutrients for the nerve cells.

The function of the spinal cord is to provide communication between the brain and all parts of the body. It is also involved with reflex actions.

Conditions associated with the central nervous system

Cerebral palsy

Cerebral palsy can be caused by abnormal brain development or birth-related brain injury. Some children suffer only the slightest of disability, others are almost totally disabled. There is often difficultly in walking and speech can be affected.

Epilepsy

Epilepsy is a disorder of the brain. Sufferers may experience 'absences' or 'seizures' (also known as petit mal and grand mal). An absence is when a person experiences momentary lapses of attention and perhaps a little abnormal movement. The seizures, or convulsions, are caused by abnormal electrical activity in the brain. Often there is no obvious cause, but in some cases the fits are due to scars on the brain from surgery or injury. Some sufferers find that flickering fluorescent lights or television screens spark off a fit. Certain essential oils may provoke fits in epileptics.

Meningitis

Meningitis is inflammation of the meninges and can be due to a bacterial or viral infection. Symptoms include stiffness in the neck, fever and headache. In severe cases, meningitis can also cause paralysis, coma and death.

Peripheral nervous system

The peripheral nervous system is concerned with all nerves situated outside the central nervous system, which includes:

- **motor nerves**, which carry nerve impulses from the brain, through the spinal cord to the skeletal muscle, glands and smooth muscular tissue to stimulate them into carrying out their work

- **sensory nerves**, which carry nerve impulses from sensory nerve endings in organs such as the skin, and transmit the impulse to the brain and spinal cord

- **mixed nerves**, which consist of motor and sensory nerves

- **interneurones**, which carry nerve impulses from sensory neurones to motor neurones. They are only found in the brain and spinal cord.

Task 7.3

Jayne has slightly burnt her finger. Which types of nerve are responsible for informing her brain of this injury? ....

Andy has spotted some money on the floor. He bends down to pick it up. Which types of nerve are responsible for the action of picking up the money?

....

Cranial nerves

There are 12 pairs of cranial nerves that originate from the brain inside the skull. They supply the muscles and sensory organs (such as the eyes and skin) of the head and neck.

Cranial nerves include ① **abducent**, ② **auditory**, ③ **facial**, ④ **glosso-pharyngeal**, ⑤ **hypoglossal**, ⑥ **oculomotor**, ⑦ **olfactory**, ⑧ **optic**, ⑨ **trochlear**, ⑩ **trigeminal**, ⑪ **accessory**, ⑫ **vagus**.

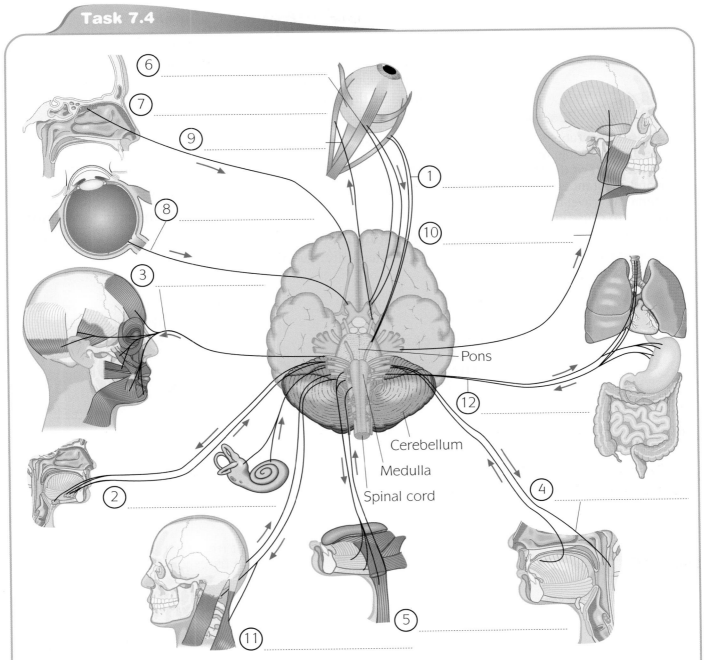

Figure 7.5 *Cranial nerves*

Label the diagram in Figure 7.5 using the information above. Use yellow to colour the nerves and brown for the brain and spinal cord.

Sense organs and receptors

The five sense organs are the eyes, ears, nose, skin and tongue. Each sense organ contains a **receptor**, which is a group of cells that are sensitive to a stimulus, such as sound or cold. Information is received by the brain from the stimulus in the form of electrical impulses (messages).

- The **eyes** contain light receptors known as rods and cones.
- The **ear** is a sense organ which contains sound receptors.
- The **nose** contains taste and smell receptors.
- The **skin** contains pressure, touch and temperature receptors.
- The **tongue** contains taste receptors which detect foods that are bitter, salty, sweet or sour.

Note

The Eustachian tube connects the middle ear with the upper part of the throat. Harmful substances such as bacteria can travel through this tube to cause infection in the middle ear.

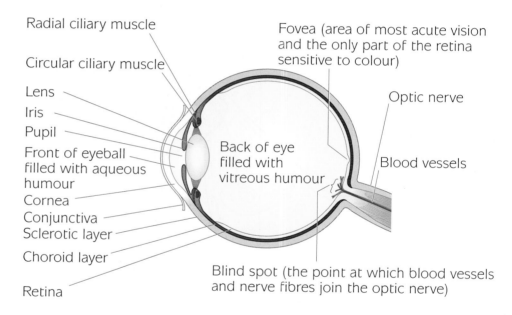

Figure 7.6 *The eye*

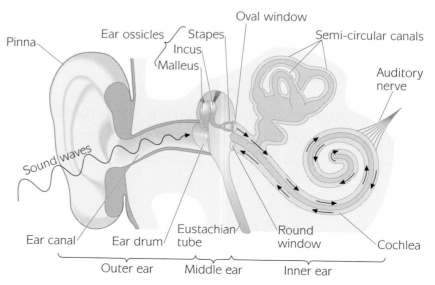

Figure 7.7 *The ear*

Spinal nerves

There are 31 pairs of spinal nerves that originate from the spinal cord and emerge between the vertebrae. The nerves are either sensory, motor or mixed (containing both types). The spinal nerves are named according to the region of the spinal cord from which they emerge (Figure 7.8). There are:

- eight pairs of cervical nerves
- 12 pairs of thoracic nerves
- five pairs of lumbar nerves
- five pairs of sacral nerves
- one pair of coccygeal nerves.

Each spinal nerve divides into branches, forming groups of nerves called **plexuses**. They are named after the vertebrae to which they connect. The main plexuses are:

- the **cervical plexus** in the neck, which supplies the skin and muscles of the head, the neck and the upper part of the shoulders and chest
- the **brachial plexus**, at the top of the shoulder, which supplies the whole of the shoulders and arm

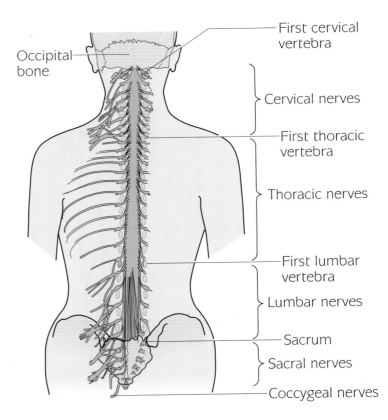

Figure 7.8 *The spinal cord and spinal nerves*

Note

The sciatic nerves are the longest nerves of the body and arise from the sacral plexus. They run down the back of each leg from the pelvis to the knees, and give branches to the lower legs and feet. They carry messages to and from all parts of the leg.

- the **thoracic plexus**, between the upper back and the waist, which supplies the chest muscles and most of the abdominal wall

- the **lumbar plexuses**, between the waist and the hip, which supply the lower part of the abdominal wall and part of the leg

- the **sacral plexuses**, at the base of the abdomen, which supply the buttock and some leg muscles

- the **coccygeal plexus**, on the back of the pelvic cavity, which supplies the muscles and skin of the pelvic area.

The nerves of the body are shown in Figure 7.9.

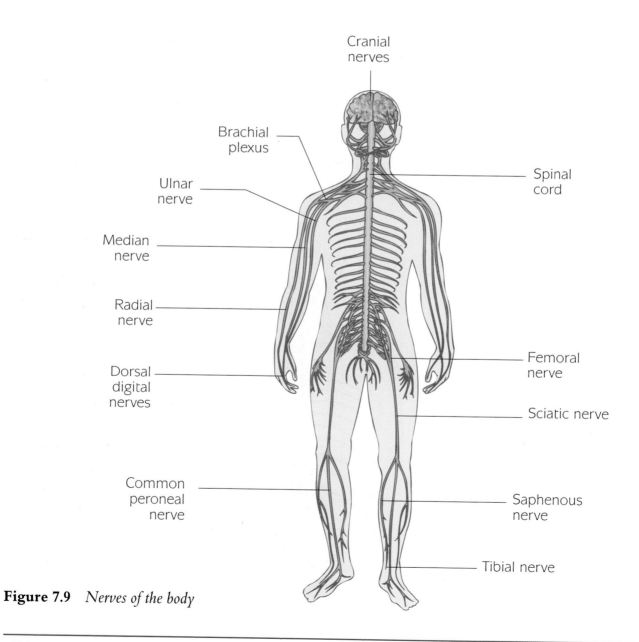

Figure 7.9   *Nerves of the body*

Reflex action

Normally nerve impulses are sent to the brain and a message is sent back, but this could take long enough for a serious injury to occur. So a **reflex action** protects the body from danger. An example of a reflex action would be the quick removal of the hands from a hot plate to prevent the hands from being burnt.

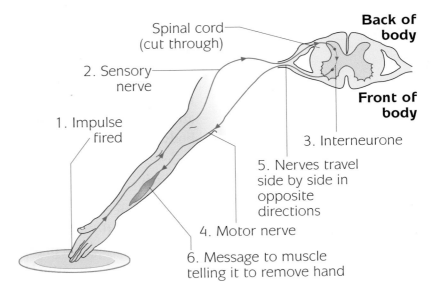

Figure 7.10   *The reflex arc*

The **reflex arc** is shown in Figure 7.10:

1   Reflex actions depend on an impulse being fired from a sensory organ (in this case pain receptors in the fingers).

2   Impulses are carried from sensory organs through sensory nerves. (Sensory nerves enter the back of the spinal cord, called the **dorsal root**.)

3   Impulses are passed from sensory nerves to interneurones.

4   Impulses pass from interneurones to motor nerves. (Motor nerves emerge from the front of the spinal cord, called the **ventral root**.)

5   Usually, motor and sensory nerves travel side-by-side through the body, although the impulses travel in opposite directions.

6   An impulse passes through the motor nerves to the muscles in the hand that had responded to the stimulus (the hot plate). The hands will then release the plate.

The reflex action ensures that the body can act quickly. Nerve impulses also travel to the brain so that it is aware of what is happening.

Conditions associated with the peripheral nervous system

Bell's palsy

Bell's palsy is inflammation of the facial nerve, often caused by injury or infection. It causes facial paralysis, although it is usually temporary.

Motor neurone disease

Motor neurone disease (MND) is a condition in which spinal nerves and motor neurones are destroyed. The main symptoms are weakness and atrophy (wasting) of all the muscles in the body.

Neuritis

Neuritis affects the peripheral nerves after they leave the spinal cord. It can affect one or several nerves. The nerves become inflamed maybe due to infection or injury. It is a painful condition and can cause loss of use of the body parts supplied by the affected nerves.

Autonomic nervous system

You can blink or move your fingers at will, but you cannot voluntarily control your heart rate or how fast your stomach digests food. The autonomic nervous system controls the involuntary movements of smooth and cardiac muscle, and of the glands, and is part of the peripheral nervous system.

The autonomic nervous system is connected to the blood vessels and the organs in the body by nerves. It is controlled by the medulla oblongata and hypothalamus, which receive impulses from the central nervous system.

The autonomic nervous system has two parts: the **sympathetic** and **parasympathetic nervous systems**, which have opposite effects. Each organ has a sympathetic and parasympathetic nerve supply:

- The **sympathetic nerves** are responsible for actions in time of stress and are made of a network of interlaced nerves or plexuses.

In reflexology, the solar plexus reflex helps to calm and relax the whole nervous system. The solar plexus is part of the autonomic nervous system and consists of sympathetic and parasympathetic nerve cells. It is a large network of nerves that controls the functioning of many organs. It is found in the abdomen at the level of the last thoracic and first lumbar vertebrae.

♦ The **parasympathetic nerves** control everyday bodily activities such as digestion and urination. They are directed towards relaxation and restorative processes. The heart rate slows, blood pressure drops and the digestive system becomes active.

In an emergency, such as when we feel threatened, the sympathetic nervous system has immediate effects on the body. Sympathetic nerves stimulate the adrenal glands to produce the hormone adrenalin. The hormone is distributed quickly by the blood and stimulates organs into greater activity. When the emergency is over the parasympathetic system returns the body to its normal state (Table 7.1).

Table 7.1 *Sympathetic and parasympathetic responses*

Part of body affected	Sympathetic stimulation	Effect	Parasympathetic stimulation
Heart	Increases heart rate	More oxygen supplied to tissues	Slows heart rate down
Coronary blood vessels	Dilate	Heart obtains more oxygen	Constrict
Skeletal muscles	Blood vessels in muscles widen	Provide more nutrients and oxygen	No effect
Bronchi/bronchioles in lungs	Dilates	More air breathed in, so more oxygen obtained	Constricts
Bladder	Relaxes wall and closes sphincter muscles	Hopefully prevents urination	Contracts bladder and opens sphincter to allow urination
Digestive system	Reduces peristalsis (wave-like contractions of food pipe)	Digestion is stopped	Increases peristalsis
Adrenal glands	Causes release of adrenalin and noradrenalin	Fight or flight	No effect
Liver	Causes conversion of glycogen to glucose	Extra glucose for tissues	Causes conversion of glucose to glycogen
Salivary glands of saliva	Decreases secretion of saliva	Dry mouth	Stimulates production of saliva
Arterioles/skin	Constricts arterioles, so less blood flows near skin surface	Skin may look pale	No effect
Sweat glands	Stimulate	Increased secretion of sweat	No effect
Eye	Dilates pupil	Vision is improved	Constricts pupil

Indicate which nerves, sympathetic or parasympathetic, are responsible for the following effects.

Effect	Nerve type
Dilation of pupils	....
Dilation of bronchi	....
Stimulation of sweat glands	....
Slowing of heart rate	....
Increased peristalsis	....
Decreased saliva production	....
Constriction of coronary blood vessels	....
Raising of glucose levels by promoting conversion of glycogen to glucose in the liver	....

Conditions associated with the autonomic nervous system

Raynaud's disease

The cause is unknown, but there is an overstimulation of the sympathetic nerves which causes blood vessels to constrict within the fingers and toes. Therefore, blood-flow is reduced and the fingers become cold. There is also tingling, burning and numbness in the affected parts.

Anxiety attack

Usually the parasympathetic nerves balance the action of the sympathetic nerves, but when we are stressed the sympathetic nerves dominate. This results in the excess release of adrenalin. Many symptoms can be experienced by a sufferer during an anxiety or panic attack, including difficulty in breathing, churning stomach, dizziness, nausea and racing heart. It can be so distressing that the sufferer may think they are going to die.

Neuralgia

Neuralgia causes brief bouts of throbbing or stabbing pain, which is often severe and sometimes shoots along the pathway of affected nerves. It is caused by irritation or damage to a nerve and is a symptom of migraine or shingles.

Parkinson's disease

This condition results from the loss of dopamine, a chemical messenger, produced in the part of the brain that controls movement. It causes muscular rigidity, tremor and slowness of movement.

Myalgic encephalomyelitis

Myalgic encephalomyelitis (ME) is a condition also known as chronic fatigue syndrome (CFS). Many cases of ME develop after suffering from a viral infection, such as glandular fever and flu. Symptoms include severe fatigue after exercise and there is also muscle weakness and pain. There may also be poor concentration, depression, disturbed sleep and mood swings.

The endocrine system

8

The nervous and endocrine systems work together to control the functions of all the body's systems. The endocrine system consists of glands situated throughout the body. The endocrine glands are ductless and secrete (release) chemical messengers called **hormones** directly into the bloodstream. Like nerves, they carry messages from one part of the body to another. The hormones are carried in the bloodstream and only affect certain cells, called **target cells**, in which they produce a response.

The trigger needed for the glands to secrete their hormones may be a nerve impulse, a chemical change in the blood or another hormone passing by that influences its release. Although minute amounts of hormones are produced by endocrine glands, they can have powerful effects upon the body.

The endocrine glands consist of the ① **pituitary gland**, ② **pineal gland**, ③ **thyroid gland**, ④ **parathyroid gland**, ⑤ **thymus**, ⑥ **adrenal glands**, ⑦ **pancreas**, ⑧ **ovaries** and ⑨ **testes**.

THE PITUITARY GLAND

The pituitary gland is situated in the middle of the brain, just behind the nose, and is about the size of a pea. It is attached by a stalk to the **hypothalamus**. The hypothalamus is made up of nerve tissue, so this stalk is where the nervous system meets the endocrine system. The hypothalamus controls many bodily activities, such as the heart rate and emptying of the bladder. It also controls the pituitary gland by stimulating, or interfering with, the release of hormones from it. Emotions such as joy and anger, as well as long-term stress, influence the endocrine system through the hypothalamus.

The pituitary gland is called the master gland because it releases several hormones that control most of the other endocrine glands, such as the ovaries, testes, thyroid gland and adrenal glands. It secretes hormones that affect growth, kidney function, delivery of babies and milk production.

> **Note**
>
> Nerves transmit their messages instantly, unlike hormones, which take longer to bring about their responses. Some hormones act within seconds, while others can take several hours or even years.

> **Note**
>
> Even a slight imbalance in the production of a hormone can result in a disorder. If too much hormone is produced, it is termed **hypersecretion**. Too little hormone is known as **hyposecretion**.

> **Fact!**
>
> Emotions such as joy and anger, as well as chronic stress, influence the endocrine system through the hypothalamus.

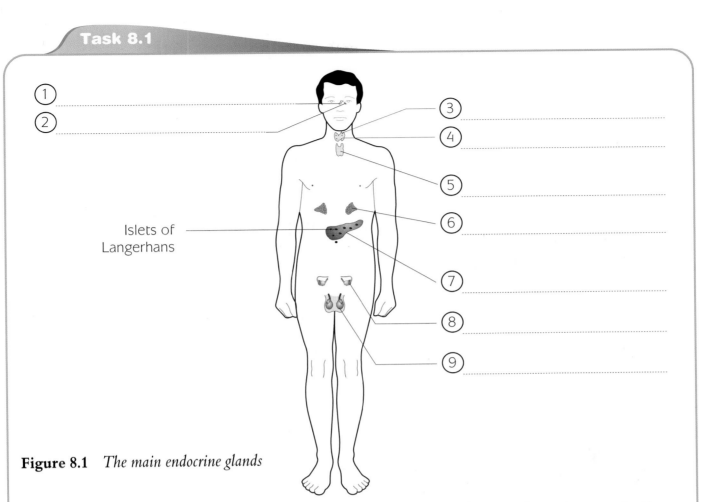

① ....

② ....

③ ....

④ ....

⑤ ....

⑥ ....

⑦ ....

⑧ ....

⑨ ....

Islets of
Langerhans

Figure 8.1 *The main endocrine glands*

Label the diagram in Figure 8.1 matching the numbers to the numbered terms in the text on page 142. Use this key to colour the endocrine glands:

Unshaded – pituitary and pineal glands
Red – thyroid and parathyroid
Green – thymus

Yellow – adrenal glands
Brown – pancreas
Orange – ovaries and testes.

The pituitary gland consists of two parts: the anterior and posterior lobes.

The anterior lobe

The anterior lobe is controlled by the hypothalamus. The following hormones are secreted by the anterior lobe (numbers refer to Task 8.2 on page 145):

① **adrenocorticotrophic hormone** (ACTH), which controls the activity of the adrenal cortex of the adrenal gland. The adrenal glands are found above each kidney

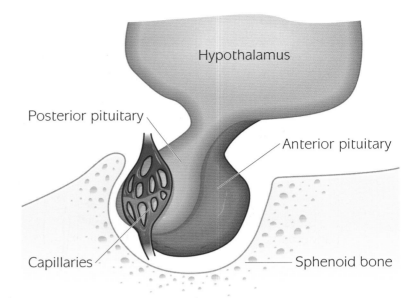

Figure 8.2 *The pituitary gland*

② **thyroid-stimulating hormone** (TSH), which controls the activity of the thyroid gland in the neck

③ **growth hormone**, sometimes called somatotropin, which controls the growth of the skeleton, muscles, connective tissues and organs such as the kidneys and liver

④ **prolactin**, which is responsible for stimulating milk production in the breasts. It has a direct effect on the breasts after pregnancy

⑤ **melanocyte-stimulating hormone** (MSH), which increases skin pigmentation by stimulating the release of melanin granules in melanocytes. The reason for this hormone is unknown.

Two **gonadotrophic hormones** control the ovaries in females and the testes in males:

⑥ **follicle-stimulating hormone** (FSH), which:
– in women stimulates the development of ova (eggs) in the ovaries and stimulates the ovaries to produce the hormone oestrogen
– in men stimulates the testes to produce sperm

⑦ **luteinising hormone** (LH), which:
– in women stimulates release of the egg from the ovary (ovulation) and production of progesterone by the ovary
– in men stimulates the testes to make the hormone testosterone.

The posterior lobe

The posterior lobe of the pituitary is controlled by nervous system stimulation of nerve cells within the hypothalamus. It releases two hormones:

⑧ **Antidiuretic hormone** (ADH) regulates water balance in the body by controlling the amount of water in urine. The hormone causes water to be returned back (reabsorption) into the blood circulation by the kidneys rather than being lost as urine. On a hot day, sweating increases and so water is lost. The body needs to hold on to as much water as it can. ADH is released, causing the kidneys to reabsorb water back into the bloodstream rather than passing it to the bladder to be excreted from the body. This results in the production of a decreased amount of urine, which will be more concentrated.

⑨ **Oxytocin** is responsible for the release of milk from the breast during suckling and for contracting the uterus during labour and after birth. Commercial preparations of oxytocin can be given to assist in childbirth.

Note

Alcohol interferes with the release of ADH from the pituitary gland. Therefore, drinking alcohol leads to an increase in the urine produced and so a person will need to urinate more frequently. Drinking a great deal of alcohol can lead to dehydration, which is largely responsible for the headache the following morning.

Task 8.2

Complete the table below. The numbers correspond to the numbered terms on pages 143–5.

Endocrine gland	Hormone released		Target organ affected	Controls or stimulates production of . . .
Anterior pituitary	①	....	....	....
Anterior pituitary	②	....	....	....
Anterior pituitary	③	....	....	....
Anterior pituitary	④	....	....	....
Anterior pituitary	⑤	....	....	....
Anterior pituitary	⑥	....	....	....
Anterior pituitary	⑦	....	....	....
Posterior pituitary	⑧	....	....	....
Posterior pituitary	⑨	....	....	....

Conditions associated with the pituitary gland

Giantism

If too much growth hormone is produced during childhood, an abnormal increase in the length of the bones will result. The long bones grow and the person becomes very tall.

Dwarfism

If too little growth hormone is produced in a young person, bone growth will slow down and other organs will also fail to grow. The person may only grow to 1–1.25 m tall. Children can be treated with growth hormone to prevent this.

Acromegaly

If too much growth hormone is produced in adulthood, it can lead to a condition called acromegaly (ak'-roe-meg'-ah-lee) in which there is bone thickening and gradual enlargement of the hands, feet, jaws, ears and nose.

Diabetes insipidus

Diabetes insipidus is associated with the posterior pituitary gland. It is either due to the gland not being able to release ADH, or the kidneys not being able to respond to it. Symptoms include large quantities of urine, dehydration and thirst.

THE PINEAL GLAND

The pineal (pin'-ee-al) gland is situated in the brain and releases a hormone called **melatonin**. More melatonin is released when a person is in darkness and this results in sleepiness. In bright sunlight, less melatonin is produced, so there is a lack of sleepiness. During sleep, the melatonin level is high and then decreases to a low level again before awakening. Thus melatonin helps to control body rhythms.

Condition associated with the pineal gland

Seasonal affective disorder

Seasonal affective disorder (SAD) is a type of depression that affects some people during the winter months when the days are short and the amount of daylight is decreased. The cause is thought to be overproduction of melatonin. Special light boxes that mimic sunlight are used to help sufferers.

THE THYROID

The thyroid is made up of two lobes and is found in front of the throat, just below the voice box. It produces the hormone **thyroxine**, which:

- Controls the body's metabolism and affects all tissues of the body. **Metabolism** is the sum of all the chemical processes going on inside the body, especially the conversion of glucose into energy by the cells – in other words, the burning of calories to provide energy for the body. Thyroxine helps to control how energetic a person is by stimulating cells to burn more or less glucose.

- Has a major influence on the development of the body mentally and physically after birth.

Another hormone released by the thyroid is called **T3** (triiodothyronin). It is essential for normal growth and metabolism.

Iodine is needed by the thyroid to produce its hormones. The body obtains iodine from the food we eat.

Conditions associated with the thyroid

Goitre

This is the result of lack of iodine and causes the thyroid gland to enlarge.

Hyperthyroidism

Overproduction of thyroxine can result in hyperthyroidism, also known as **overactive thyroid**. This causes the metabolism to speed up so that the sufferer loses weight, has a fast heart beat and increased sweating, and also develops bulging eyes because of the swelling of tissues behind them. This is a dangerous condition, which needs medical treatment.

Hypothyroidism

Undersecretion of thyroxine causes hypothyroidism, also known as **underactive thyroid**. This causes the metabolism to slow down so that the sufferer puts on weight and becomes lethargic. The hair becomes dry and brittle and there may be some loss of hair. The skin appears thickened, coarse and dry. The circulation may be poor so the sufferer feels the cold more than normal. This condition also needs medical treatment.

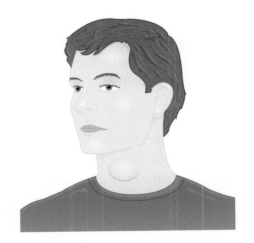

Figure 8.3 *Goitre*

THE PARATHYROID

The four tiny parathyroid glands can be found embedded on the back of the thyroid gland. They produce the hormone **parathormone**.

The parathyroids are sensitive to the levels of calcium in the blood. Calcium is important as it is needed for muscle contraction, transmission of nerve impulses and blood clotting. The main function of parathormone is to control calcium levels in the blood to maintain normal limits:

- If calcium levels become very high, **calcitonin** is released from the thyroid gland. This hormone quickly helps to prevent removal of calcium from the bones.

- If calcium levels are low, parathormone will cause calcium to be taken from bones, decrease the rate at which calcium is lost from the urine and increase absorption of calcium from the small intestine to increase levels within the blood.

Conditions associated with the parathyroid

Hypersecretion

Overproduction of parathormone causes an increased amount of calcium in the blood. It may cause excess calcium to be lost from the bones, leading to brittle bones that fracture easily (**osteoporosis**).

The hormone **oestrogen**, produced by the ovaries, interferes with the release of parathormone. After the menopause the oestrogen levels in the body decrease. This means that parathormone is no longer inhibited, so excess calcium may be taken from the bones, which can also lead to osteoporosis.

Hyposecretion

Undersecretion of parathormone can lead to a deficiency of calcium in the body. As calcium is needed for muscle contraction, it can lead to a condition known as **tetany**, in which the muscles become stiff and go into spasm.

THE THYMUS

The thymus gland is situated in the thorax (chest region) behind the sternum. It is made up of lymphoid tissue. In an infant it is large, but after puberty it begins to waste away. The thymus is thought to act as a brake on sexual development until puberty. It releases hormones, one of which is called **thymosin**. Thymosin is involved with the production of lymphocytes, which help fight against viruses and other infections in the body.

Task 8.3

Complete the table below.

Endocrine gland	Hormone released	Effect
Pineal	....	....
	....	....
Thyroid	....	....
	....	....
Parathyroid	....	....
	....	....
Thymus	....	....
	....	....

THE ADRENAL GLANDS

The adrenal glands are found on top of each kidney. They are made of two parts: the cortex and the medulla. The cortex is the outside and the medulla the inner part of the gland.

Adrenal cortex

The adrenal cortex is essential to life and plays an important role in states of stress. It is known that the adrenal cortex releases over 50 hormones. All of these hormones are steroids and are produced from a fatty substance called **cholesterol**. They are grouped into three categories: sex corticoids, glucocorticoids and mineral corticoids, according to the type of action in which they are involved.

① Sex corticoids

These help control the changes in males and females during puberty. The female sex hormones **oestrogen** and male hormones **androgens** are produced in small amounts from this gland.

Fact!

Androgen levels rise in women during puberty, pregnancy and the menopause.

Conditions associated with sex corticoids

Hirsutism

Oestrogen and androgens are produced in both males and females. Men produce more androgens than women. If a woman is particularly sensitive to androgens, excess hair may develop in the male pattern, e.g. on the chin. This is called hirsutism. Androgen levels rise in women during puberty, pregnancy and the menopause.

Virilism

Virilism is a condition in which there is an oversecretion of androgens in a female. The increased amount of androgens causes the woman to become masculine. Symptoms develop such as receding hairline, increased growth of body and facial hair, the voice deepens and the menstrual cycle stops.

Gynaecomastia

This is a condition affecting males only and is mostly temporary. It is due to increased oestrogen levels in the body. The sufferer develops excessive growth of one breast or both.

② Glucocorticoids

The glucocorticoids help to regulate nutrient levels within the blood. They help the body process food that we eat and turn it into energy. One main glucocorticoid is called **cortisol**, also known as **hydrocortisone**. Stress, anger, fright or rapidly falling sugar levels can cause ACTH (adrenocorticotrophic hormone) to be released from the anterior pituitary. This stimulates the release of cortisol by the adrenal glands.

Cortisol has several functions:

- It provides more rapid breakdown of glycogen into glucose for extra energy during a crisis or an increased need. This raises sugar levels in the blood to ensure that cells have sufficient glucose for energy.

- **Adrenalin** is quickly released from the adrenal medulla whenever danger threatens. Cortisol is released a little while later and prepares the body for the after-effects of danger. Cortisol helps reduce the feelings of pain, which is why people who are severely injured may feel no pain until some time later.

- It affects the metabolism by increasing the use of protein and fats as a source of energy in the body. Cortisol causes proteins to be broken down into amino acids. The amino acids can be converted into glucose by the liver. Cortisol also acts on fats, which are broken down into fatty acids. The glucose and fatty acids are used by the body as sources of energy.

Fact!

Cortisol helps reduce the feelings of pain, which is why people who are severely injured may feel no pain until some time later.

- It helps to control body rhythms. Cortisol levels are highest between 6 a.m. and 9 a.m. and trigger waking from sleep. The levels are at their lowest between midnight and 3 a.m. and so promote sleepiness.

- It has anti-inflammatory actions, inhibiting cells from taking part in inflammatory responses. Cortisol is mimicked by corticosteroid drugs, which have a huge range of uses and are used to treat inflammatory and allergic conditions such as asthma, hay fever, psoriasis and arthritis.

③ *Mineral corticoids*

Mineral corticoids help to maintain the right balance of the minerals such as sodium (salt) and potassium in the body. One of the mineral corticoids is called **aldosterone** and is released if sodium levels drop in the body, e.g. through sweating a lot. Aldosterone ensures that the sodium is passed back into the blood from the kidneys and not excreted in the urine; this helps to increase sodium levels. Oversecretion of aldosterone causes increased levels of sodium, which can lead to fluid retention (**oedema**).

Conditions associated with glucocorticoids and mineral corticoids

Addison's disease
This results from abnormally low levels of aldosterone and cortisol. Symptoms include low blood glucose levels, low levels of sodium (salt) in the blood, inability to use fat and protein for energy, low blood pressure and excessive urination.

Cushing's syndrome
Cushing's syndrome is caused by oversecretion of cortisol and aldosterone. The symptoms include a moon-shaped face, wasting of muscle tissue, high blood levels of glucose, high blood pressure and excess fat tissue on the trunk of the body.

Adrenal medulla

The adrenal medulla produces hormones called ④ **adrenalin** and ⑤ **noradrenalin**, which together prepare the body for action, known as the **fight or flight response**. In response to stress, such as being chased by a bull, the hypothalamus sends a message via sympathetic nerves to the adrenal glands. Adrenalin is released and is distributed quickly by the blood.

Adrenalin has the following effects:

- The heart beats stronger and faster, which increases blood pressure.

- The arteries supplying the skin and internal organs constrict and so blood flow decreases. However, the blood flow increases in skeletal muscle so that the extra oxygen and glucose can help to provide extra energy. This is why we can look pale in an emergency.

- Adrenalin also increases the breakdown of glycogen to glucose in the liver. This ensures that there is a ready supply for the muscles.

- The airway passages dilate (widen), allowing air to move in and out of the lungs with greater ease.

- Adrenalin also stimulates ACTH, so that glucocorticoids are released, and TSH to increase the metabolism to help prepare the body for action.

Adrenalin may be injected to restart a heart when it stops during a heart attack. It can also be given to someone suffering an asthma attack.

Fact!

Adrenalin may be injected to restart a heart when it stops during a heart attack. It can also be given to someone suffering an asthma attack.

Task 8.4

Complete the table below. The numbers correspond to the numbered terms in the text on pages 149–51.

Endocrine gland	Hormone released	Effect
Adrenal cortex	①	....
	....	....
Adrenal cortex	②	....
	....	....
Adrenal cortex	③	....
	....	....
Adrenal medulla	④	....
	....	....
Adrenal medulla	⑤	....
	....	....

Carbohydrates are made up of many sugar molecules, mostly glucose. Eating carbohydrate food means a rise of sugar in the blood. Vigorous exercise causes a lot of glucose to be used by muscles, which lowers the sugar levels in the blood.

The **islets of Langerhans** in the pancreas are sensitive to sugar levels in the body. To maintain the balance of sugar in the blood, the islets of Langerhans release hormones:

- When blood sugar levels are too high, the hormone ① **insulin** is released. Insulin causes the liver and muscles to store glucose in the form of glycogen (lots of glucose molecules joined together). This helps to bring the blood sugar levels down.

- If sugar levels are too low in the blood, the hormone ② **glucagon** is released. It causes the liver and muscles to release glucose into the bloodstream to help restore levels.

Condition associated with the pancreas

Diabetes mellitus

Diabetes mellitus is a disease caused *either* by the pancreas producing insufficient amounts of insulin *or* by the tissues not responding to insulin. This results in the sugar (glucose) level in the blood rising too high, which leads to the symptoms and complications of diabetes such as tiredness and thirst.

Insulin is needed by the body to allow glucose to enter into the cells. Without insulin the cells cannot process the glucose to produce energy, which may result in fats being broken down to provide energy instead. The breakdown of fats could result in a build-up of chemicals called **ketones** in the bloodstream, which are produced by the liver. A build-up of ketones may lead to illness.

There are two types of diabetes mellitus:

- **Type one** is often called **insulin-dependent diabetes** and mostly develops in people under the age of 20. This type is more serious and is often caused by the production of little or no insulin. With this type, it is essential to have insulin treatment to survive. The symptoms develop quickly and include dehydration, excessive thirst, increased urination, weight loss, vomiting, drowsiness, weakness and finally coma.

- **Type two** is more common and often affects people over the age of 35 who are overweight. It is also called **maturity-onset**

diabetes mellitus. This type usually develops from the reduced ability of the tissues to respond to insulin, although insulin is still being produced. Type two diabetes can often be controlled by diet, exercise and weight loss. The symptoms are similar to type one, but they develop gradually and are less severe. Diabetic coma does not occur with type two.

Treatment for diabetes rapidly restores health to normal. However, poorly controlled diabetes over a long period of time can cause the following problems:

- The tissues can become damaged and waste away; for example, the skin may become paper-thin. There may also be skin infections such as spots and boils.

- Eye diseases such as diabetic retinopathy can develop and in a few people can lead to blindness. Diabetic retinopathy is caused by blood leaking from damaged capillaries.

- High blood pressure is more common in diabetics. It can lead to capillary damage in the kidneys, causing swollen ankles, fatigue and the build-up of urea which is a harmful waste product in the blood.

- Damage to nerves (neuritis) can lead to a loss of sensation in the legs but mainly affects the feet. An example of this is of a diabetic who, while walking, did not realise that there was a golf ball inside one shoe.

- Problems arise because the diabetic may be unaware of injury to the feet. The injuries may be further aggravated by poor circulation; therefore healing is poor, which can lead to ulcers and infection. This can become serious and may even lead to amputation.

- Hardening and narrowing of the arteries is more common in diabetics. This can cause poor circulation in the legs and feet. It can also contribute to heart attack and stroke.

Diabetes mellitus can be treated with insulin injections. The insulin passes directly into the bloodstream and so is effective straight away. Occasionally, diabetics can give themselves too much insulin, which results in a condition called **hypoglycaemia** – an abnormally low level of sugar in the blood. The sufferer sweats, trembles, has blurred vision and lacks concentration. The behaviour of someone suffering from hypoglycaemia may be mistaken for drunkenness. A sweet snack, such as fruit juice or a small chocolate bar, is needed to raise the sugar levels in the blood.

The ovaries are a pair of almond-shaped organs found within the female pelvis, one on either side of the womb. They produce the female hormones oestrogen and progesterone, which are responsible for all female secondary sexual characteristics such as breasts, a female body shape and **ova** (egg) production:

③ **Oestrogen** causes the lining of the uterus to thicken and grow during a menstrual cycle. It also stimulates the release of an egg from the ovary.

④ **Progesterone** maintains the lining of the uterus. When the levels of progesterone fall, the lining then breaks down and is shed in the menstrual flow.

Effects of hormones at puberty

Puberty in girls normally begins at around 11 years old. When a girl reaches puberty, her ovaries grow up to 10 times larger. As the ovaries grow, they release the hormone oestrogen, which is responsible for the bodily changes at puberty such as female curves and the growth of the breasts. After an egg is released (**ovulation**), the ovaries release progesterone to prepare the body for possible pregnancy. If the egg is not fertilised, the ovaries stop producing progesterone and the menstrual period follows.

Androgen levels in girls also increase at puberty, causing axillary (under the armpit) and pubic hair growth. Androgens are also a main cause of acne by causing inflammation of the sebaceous glands.

Effect of hormones in pregnancy

During pregnancy there is an increase in hormonal activity (see Chapter 10). Sometimes, excess androgens can be produced, resulting in excess hair growth. It is usually only temporary and returns to normal after the baby is born.

Large brown patches can appear on the skin during pregnancy, especially the face. These are known as **chloasma**. High levels of oestrogen and progesterone are thought to be the cause.

Effect of hormones at the menopause

The menopause usually begins between the ages of 45 and 55. The ovaries decrease in size and no longer respond to the gonadotrophic hormones of the anterior pituitary gland. Oestrogen levels therefore decrease. Oestrogen is thought to help protect the bones. The decrease in oestrogen levels may therefore lead to **osteoporosis**, a condition in which the bones become brittle and fracture easily.

The low levels of oestrogen also cause the menstrual cycle to become irregular and gradually stop. The breasts start to shrink and there is thinning of the axillary and pubic hair. During the menopause increased levels of androgens can cause excess facial and body hair.

Symptoms of the menopause

Symptoms of the menopause include hot flushes, headaches, depression, insomnia, fatigue and inability to concentrate, and the skin and hair can become dry. Many of the symptoms of the menopause, especially hot flushes, appear to be a result of altered function of the hypothalamus. **Endorphins** are the body's own mood-lifting and pain-relieving hormones and are critical to the proper functioning of the hypothalamus. Exercise and acupuncture can enhance endorphin output.

To help with the symptoms of the menopause, women are often treated with **hormone replacement therapy** (HRT), which consists of oestrogen and progesterone. HRT can give relief from menopausal symptoms, including hot flushes, and can help with the laying down of new bone to protect against the development of osteoporosis. The oestrogen also helps to keep the skin and hair in good condition. HRT can slightly increase the risk of developing breast cancer.

A healthy diet, exercise and lifestyle factors have been shown to offer identical benefits of HRT and without the risks. Fat produces oestrogen and as the oestrogen levels decrease during the menopause, body fat becomes an alternative manufacturing plant for making oestrogen. Oestrogen can help protect the older woman from osteoporosis so it is advisable to have a diet which includes some fat.

THE TESTES

Testes are found in the groin area of the male in a sac called the **scrotum**. The testes produce the hormone ⑤ **testosterone**, which is responsible for all male secondary sexual characteristics at puberty, such as body hair, deep voice and muscle development.

The testes also contain fine tubes in which sperm are produced when stimulated by follicle-stimulating hormone.

The production of testosterone from the testes decreases with age, although many older men still produce active sperm in normal numbers.

Task 8.5

Complete the table below. The numbers correspond to the numbered terms in the text on pages 153–6.

Endocrine gland	Hormone released	Effect
Pancreas	①	....
Pancreas	②	....
Ovaries	③	....
Ovaries	④	....
Testes	⑤	....

The digestive system

9

Fact!

Food takes on average 24 hours to pass through the digestive tract.

The digestive system changes the food we eat into small, simple molecules that can be absorbed into the bloodstream and used by the body to produce energy or as building materials for repairing itself or growing.

DIGESTION

Task 9.1

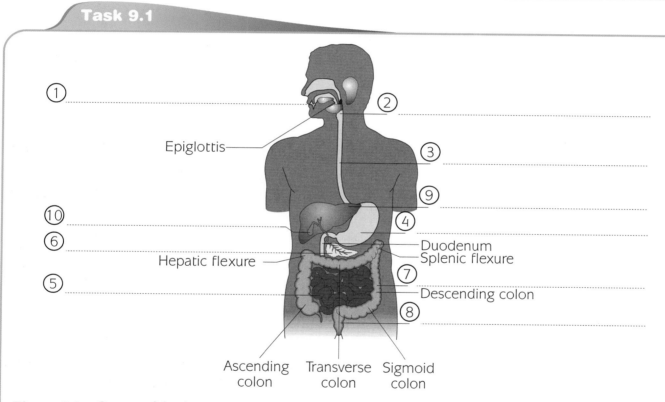

Epiglottis

①

②

③

⑨

⑩

⑥

④

Duodenum
Splenic flexure

Hepatic flexure

⑦

⑤

Descending colon

⑧

Ascending colon   Transverse colon   Sigmoid colon

Figure 9.1 *Organs of the digestive system*

Label the diagram in Figure 9.1 matching the numbers to the numbered terms in the following text. Use this key to colour the organs of the digestive system:

Pink – mouth, oesophagus, stomach, small intestine, large intestine and rectum.

Brown – liver
Green – gall bladder
Yellow – pancreas.

The **digestive tract**, also known as the **alimentary canal**, is more than 10 metres long and begins at the mouth and ends at the anus.

① Mouth

The taking of food and liquids into the mouth is called **ingestion**. The action of the teeth helps to break down the food during chewing, also called **mastication**.

There are three main pairs of salivary glands which produce saliva:

- The **parotid glands** are located in front of and below the ears, between the skin and the masseter muscle.
- The **submandibular glands** and **sublingual glands** are found below the tongue.

The saliva lubricates the food and in most people contains an enzyme called **salivary amylase**. An enzyme is a protein that speeds up chemical reactions. This enzyme begins the break down of starch in cooked foods. Starch is found in foods like bread, potatoes and grains.

Tongue

The tongue contains nerve receptors and is divided into four main areas that detect sour, salty, bitter and sweet flavours.

- Sourness and saltiness are detected by taste buds at the sides of the tongue.
- Bitterness is detected by taste buds at the back of the tongue.
- Sweetness is detected by taste buds at the front of the tongue.

Note

The adult set of teeth consists of 32 teeth.

② Pharynx

The muscles of the pharynx (throat) push the food down into the **oesophagus** (food pipe). A flap of cartilage known as the **epiglottis** prevents the food being swallowed from entering the lungs.

③ Oesophagus

This is the food pipe, which is a muscular tube leading to the stomach. The passage of food is aided by the release of mucus from the wall of the oesophagus. The food is propelled downwards towards the stomach by the process of **peristalsis**. Peristalsis is a wave of contractions occurring in the muscles of the oesophagus wall. The walls squeeze and relax to push food along the digestive tract.

④ Stomach

This is a muscular, J-shaped, bag-like organ situated on the left side of the abdominal cavity beneath the diaphragm. At either end of the stomach is a sphincter muscle which contracts and relaxes to control the movement of food in and out of the stomach. The stomach churns the food and releases gastric juices to help break it down. The gastric juices contain hydrochloric acid and enzymes such as pepsin.

- **Hydrochloric acid** kills any harmful bacteria and helps to dissolve the food.

- **Pepsin** begins the digestion of protein by breaking it down.

Substances including water, alcohol and glucose are absorbed directly into the bloodstream from the stomach. Food stays within the stomach for about five hours and leaves in a liquid form called **chyme**.

⑤ The small intestine

The small intestine is over 6 metres long and is the place where most of the nutrients are absorbed. There are three parts to the small intestine: the first part is called the **duodenum**, followed by the **jejunum** and then the **ileum**.

The inside of the small intestine is covered with millions of tiny finger-like projections called **villi**. Villi have a rich blood supply and their shape ensures a large surface area so that digested food can be absorbed quickly (Figure 9.2). The nutrients are passed into the bloodstream, with the exception of fat. Fat is absorbed directly into lymphatic capillaries called **lacteals** and so gives lymph a milky colour. The fat joins the lymphatic system before finally reaching the blood circulation.

Note

Rennin is an enzyme that curdles milk and is only found in the stomachs of infants.

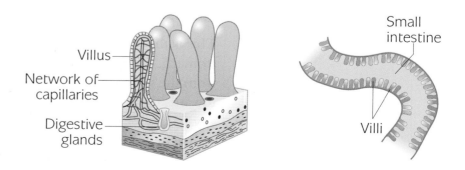

Villus
Network of capillaries
Digestive glands
Small intestine
Villi

Figure 9.2 *Villi*

Breakdown of foods

Carbohydrates such as starch and glycogen consist of long chains of glucose molecules.

- Starch digestion begins in the mouth, when salivary amylase begins breaking down the starch molecules to become the sugar **maltose**.

- In the duodenum, the enzyme **maltase** breaks down each maltose molecule to two molecules of glucose. **Sucrose**, the sugar we use in our tea, is broken down by the enzyme **sucrase** into glucose and fructose, and **lactose** (milk sugar) is broken down by the enzyme **lactase** into glucose and galactose.

Proteins are made up of smaller molecules called **amino acids**.

- Protein digestion begins in the stomach with the enzyme **pepsin**, which breaks down most proteins into smaller units called **polypeptides**.

- In the duodenum, the enzyme **trypsin,** found in the pancreatic juice, breaks down proteins and polypeptides into smaller substances called **peptides**. Peptides are broken down by enzymes to become **amino acids**:

$$\text{Protein} \xrightarrow{\text{Pepsin}} \text{Polypeptides} \xrightarrow{\text{Trypsin}} \text{Peptides} \rightarrow \text{Amino acids}$$

Organs such as the pancreas and liver also play a part in the digestion of food. The pancreas releases pancreatic juices into the duodenum and is responsible for breaking down protein, carbohydrates and fats. The liver produces **bile** which also helps to break down fats.

⑥ Pancreas

The pancreas is a gland situated behind the stomach and is about 15 cm long. As well as releasing hormones, it also produces the following enzymes:

- **trypsin**, which digests proteins and breaks them down into amino acids

- **amylase**, which continues the digestion of starch molecules into the sugar maltose

- **lipase**, which breaks down fats into fatty acids and glycerol.

The pancreas also keeps a check on the amount of glucose in the blood. If the level is too high or too low it produces hormones that stimulate the liver to adjust the balance (see Chapter 8).

⑦ Large intestine

The large intestine is also called the **colon** and is called 'large' because of its diameter, not its length. It is about 1.5 metres long and is divided into the **ascending**, **transverse** and **descending colon**. The **hepatic flexure** is found between the ascending and transverse colon and the **splenic flexure** is found between the transverse and descending colon. The **sigmoid colon** is an S-shape and ends at the sacral vertebrae.

Any remaining undigested food and fibre (roughage) is now waste matter and passes from the small intestine into the large intestine in liquid form. Any remaining nutrients and water are removed from this waste matter and reabsorbed back into the body. This results in solid faeces being formed.

The large intestine contains millions of bacteria which are useful as they produce vitamins B and K, which are absorbed and used by the body. These bacteria also have the ability to ferment some forms of carbohydrates found in foods such as onions and beans, which are not digested by the enzymes of the small intestine. This fermentation produces large quantities of a gas, termed **flatulence** when it is excessive.

⑧ Rectum

The rectum is about 13 cm long and has two sphincter muscles at the end which form the **anus**. Waste matter is expelled through the anus. This is called **elimination**.

⑨ Liver

The liver is a large organ found in the upper right corner of the abdomen and extending across to the left side. It lies below the diaphragm and is mostly protected by the ribs.

Most of the blood entering the liver passes through the **hepatic portal vein** which carries blood from the stomach, intestines, spleen, pancreas and ⑩ **gall bladder**. The blood in the portal vein carries nutrients such as glucose, amino acids (protein), vitamins and minerals.

Note

- The **ileo-caecal** (il'-ee-o-see'-kal) **valve** lies between the small and large intestine and prevents faeces going in a backwards direction.

- The **appendix** is a narrow, worm-like tube closed at one end that leads off from the large intestine and has no known function.

Note

The **sigmoid colon** is the last intestinal turn before waste is emptied into the rectum. It is an area that is worked on during a reflexology treatment.

Note

The word 'hepatic' means 'belonging to the liver'.

Fill in the gaps in the table below.

Organ	Enzyme or acid	Action
Mouth	Salivary amylase	....
Stomach	....	Kills bacteria
Stomach	Pepsin	....
Liver	Bile	....
Pancreas	....	Breaks down protein
Pancreas	Amylase	....
Pancreas	....	Breaks down fats

Fact!

The liver carries out over 500 functions in the body.

Fact!

The liver has the remarkable ability to regenerate itself if it becomes damaged. If half of the liver is cut away, it will quickly grow back to the original size.

The pear-shaped gallbladder stores **bile**, a greenish fluid produced by the liver. After food has been eaten, bile is released and travels down the **bile duct** to the duodenum where it begins to break down fats into small droplets which are easier for lipase to digest.

Functions of the liver

The functions include:

- storing and filtering the blood
- destroying bacteria and worn out red blood cells
- breaking down excess proteins into urea which is excreted in the urine
- secreting bile to help break down fat
- detoxification of harmful substances such as alcohol, paracetamol and other chemicals into safer forms
- storage of vitamins A, D, E and K, and iron
- storage of glycogen, which can be broken down into glucose and used for energy by the body when required
- converting certain nutrients into others – amino acids (protein) can be turned into lipids (fats) or glucose (sugar) if required.

Conditions associated with the digestive system

Peptic ulcers

These are areas of erosion in the lining of the stomach and are due to damage by the acidic digestive juices.

Duodenal ulcers

Duodenal ulcers are found in the duodenum. These ulcers are often linked to bacterial infection.

Cirrhosis

Cirrhosis is a liver disease caused by cell damage, and there is a gradual build-up of scarred tissue which prevents the liver from functioning normally to remove toxins from the blood. It is often due to high alcohol intake.

Jaundice

This is a symptom of various disorders including hepatitis. It refers to the yellowing of the skin and the whites of the eyes. In bile there is a pigment called **bilirubin** which gives faeces its brown colouring. If the liver is diseased or the bile ducts are blocked, the bilirubin cannot get out. Therefore, it gradually accumulates in the blood and stains the tissues giving the skin its yellow colouring.

Appendicitis

Appendicitis is inflammation of the appendix. Too much bacteria in the appendix can cause infection leading to swelling and pain. It can be dangerous if the appendix bursts, so it is removed.

Heartburn

This causes a burning pain in the foodpipe and chest. It can be due to overeating, too much alcohol, stress and pregnancy.

Hernia

- An **abdominal hernia** can occur during exercise, especially lifting a heavy weight, and puts strain on the abdominal wall. The hernia can be seen bulging through the abdominal wall and causes pain.

- A **hiatus hernia** results when part of the stomach ends up above the diaphragm as it protrudes through a space usually occupied by the oesophagus.

Note

Both anorexia and bulimia can cause lack of periods, dry flaky skin, thinning of scalp hair, tiredness, pale skin, and an excess growth of downy hair can appear on the body.

Anorexia nervosa

This is a condition in which sufferers are obsessed with not eating and have a phobia concerning body fat.

Bulimia nervosa

This involves the sufferer alternately binge-eating and vomiting or purging with laxatives and diuretics.

Irritable bowel syndrome

Irritable bowel syndrome (IBS) is a common disorder and mostly affects women. It causes recurrent pain in the abdomen with diarrhoea that often alternates with constipation. Other symptoms include a bloated abdomen, excessive wind, tiredness, nausea and headaches. Causes include stress and sensitivity to certain foods.

Diarrhoea and constipation

- **Diarrhoea** is the passing of frequent, loose, watery stools and results when the contents of the bowel pass through too quickly so there is insufficient time for the water to be absorbed. Diarrhoea can be caused by stress, eating certain foods, food poisoning or drinking too much alcohol. It is the body's way of getting rid of harmful substances in the colon.

- If the contents remain too long in the colon, too much water is withdrawn from the faeces resulting in **constipation**, which includes the passing of hard stools, often with difficulty. A common cause of constipation is lack of roughage in the diet.

Gall stones

These are stones made mostly from cholesterol and are found in the gall bladder. A stone may block the flow of bile causing inflammation. Symptoms include pain in the upper right abdomen, nausea, indigestion and jaundice.

Coeliac disease

Coeliac (cee-lee-ak) disease is caused by sensitivity to gluten and often runs in families. Gluten is found in many foods including bread. Severe stress, physical injury, infection, pregnancy or surgery may lead to symptoms developing. Symptoms include diarrhoea, abdominal pain, tiredness, anaemia, mouth ulcers and weight loss.

Diverticulitis

This is a disorder that affects the lining of the large intestine. Small pockets known **diverticuli** form in weakened areas of the wall. There is inflammation and abdominal pain, which usually occurs on the left-hand side. Other symptoms include constipation and diarrhoea. It is caused by lack of fibre in the diet.

NUTRITION

Food contains substances called **nutrients** found within five basic food groups: protein, carbohydrates, fats, vitamins and minerals. Although fibre is not nutritionally valuable, it is important for a healthy diet. All foods contain some nutrients, but hardly any food contains all of them.

For the body to remain healthy, a variety of foods need to be eaten (Table 9.1).

Fact!

As many as 70 per cent of cancers are thought to be diet related.

Table 9.1 *Food groups, good sources and their effects on the body*

Food group	Function	Good sources
Protein	Vital for growth and repair of cells	Meat, fish, eggs, milk, cheese
Carbohydrates	Provide energy for the body	Potatoes, bread, sugar, cereals, pasta
Fats	Provide energy for the body	Butter, lard, vegetable oil, cheese
Vitamins and minerals	Essential for growth and general health	Fruit and vegetables
Fibre	Helps keep the muscles of the intestines exercised, prevents constipation and provides bulk to satisfy appetite	Vegetables, fruit, cereals and wholemeal foods

Sugars

Monosaccharides are known as **single sugars** or **simple sugars**. They are small, sweet to taste and soluble in water. An example is fructose found in fruit and honey. The liver converts fructose into glucose. Glucose is very important as all the body's cells require it.

Dissaccharides are known as **double sugars**. They are small, sweet to taste and soluble in water. They are formed when two monosaccharides join together. Examples of disaccharides include lactose (the sugar found in milk) and sucrose (found in sugar).

Table 9.2 *Vitamins*

Vitamins	Best sources	Functions	Deficiency signs
Vitamin A Retinol	Fish liver oils, dairy products, liver, eggs, vegetables and fruit	Needed for normal vision, even in dim light. Required for teeth and bone formation. Helps protect against infections	Night blindness, dry, rough skin and reduced resistance to infection
Vitamin B$_1$ Thiamine	Wholegrain cereals, brown rice, wholemeal bread, nuts, eggs, fish and milk	Helps convert carbohydrate into energy	Loss of appetite, lack of concentration, muscle weakness and depression
Vitamin B$_2$ Riboflavin	Wheat bran, green, leafy vegetables, peas and beans, meat, eggs and milk	Releases energy from carbohydrates, proteins and fats, maintains healthy skin	Cracked lips, soreness of mouth and tongue, dermatitis, hair loss, blurred vision and dizziness
Vitamin B$_3$ Niacin	Wholegrain cereals, peas, beans, nuts, meat, eggs and fish	Helps to release energy from fats, glucose. Maintains healthy skin, nervous and digestive systems	Rare. Loss of appetite, weight loss, nausea, depression
Vitamin B$_5$ Pantothenic acid	Most foods, especially wholegrain cereals, wheat germ, green vegetables, nuts, eggs and fish	Helps to release energy from fats and carbohydrates, beneficial for nervous system, converts cholesterol into anti-stress hormones	Exhaustion, abdominal pain, headache, cramps, more prone to infections
Vitamin B$_6$ Pyridoxine	Most foods, wholegrain cereals, wheat germ, green vegetables nuts, eggs and fish	Needed for metabolism carbohydrates, protein and fat, production of antibodies to fight infection, healthy skin	Skin problems, cracked lips, possibly PMS, depression, and kidney stones
Vitamin B$_{12}$ Cyanocobalamin	Liver, meat, fish, pork, beef, animal products	Detoxifies cyanide brought into body by smoking and food	Pernicious anaemia, nerve damage so causes tremors, mental deterioration, menstrual disorder, pigmentation of the hands and tiredness
Vitamin C	Citrus fruits, broccoli, peppers, tomatoes	Needed for healthy bones, teeth and gums and resistance against infection and for body to absorb iron	Aches, pains, swollen gums, nose bleeds, anaemia, scurvy, haemorrhaging
Vitamin D	Fish, cod liver oil, liver, eggs, dairy products and margarine	Needed for strong bones and teeth, blood clotting, muscle and nerve function	Rickets in children, osteomalacia in adults, weakened bones, restlessness, poor muscle tone
Vitamin E	Vegetable oils, egg yolks, wheat germ, nuts, wholegrain cereals, leafy green vegetables	Slows down ageing by protecting cell membranes, needed for the formation of red blood cells	Rare. Anaemia and destruction of red blood cells

Fats

There is a lot of hidden fat in the snacks we eat (biscuits, crisps, chocolate). When the body has too much fat it is stored under the skin as adipose tissue and can be broken down to make energy if required. The body needs some fats to:

- protect the organs
- transport fat-soluble vitamins
- provide insulation and energy.

There are two main types of fat:

- **Saturated fat** is found in animal products such as meat, butter and full-fat cheese. These fats are the most damaging to health as saturated fat is converted to cholesterol by our bodies. This may cause raised levels of bad blood cholesterol, which clog up the arteries and lead to heart disease and strokes.

- **Unsaturated fats** are derived from plants. There are two kinds of unsaturated fats: monounsaturated and polyunsaturated. Monounsaturated are the healthier choice as they are said to lower bad blood cholesterol. Olive oil and rapeseed oil are good sources.

Fact!

Coconut oil and palm oil, although derived from plants, also contain saturated fats.

Table 9.3 *Minerals*

Mineral	Functions	Where it can be found
Calcium	Needed for teeth and bones; essential for blood clotting and for muscle and nerve function	Milk and other dairy products, fish and green, leafy vegetables
Phosphorus	Needed for bones, teeth and nerve and muscle function	Meat, cereal, dairy products
Potassium	Influences nerve function and muscle contraction	Fruit, vegetables and grains
Sodium	Important in fluid balance and the passing of impulses between neurones, also muscle contraction	Many foods, table salt
Magnesium	Needed for muscle and nerve function. Also bones and teeth	Nuts; whole grains, green, leafy vegetables
Iron	Part of haemoglobin which carry oxygen in red blood cells	Meat, nuts, egg yolk, dried fruit
Iodine	Needed for the production of thyroid hormones	Seafood, salt, vegetables grown in iodine-rich soils

The reproductive systems

10

The reproductive systems of men and women ensure that new human life can be created. This can only happen when a woman's ovum (egg) is fertilised by a man's sperm.

The female reproductive system consists of a uterus (womb), two Fallopian tubes and two ovaries. In the male the organs include the testes (which are protected in a sac called the scrotum), the vas deferens and the penis.

Fact!

The male reproductive organs are found outside the body cavity because the testes need to be kept a couple of degrees cooler than normal body temperature to produce fertile sperm.

The female reproductive organs are situated within the pelvic cavity – the pelvic bones help to protect them. The pelvic cavity is wider in the female than the male to allow more space for childbirth. The male reproductive organs are found outside the body cavity because the testes need to be kept a couple of degrees cooler than normal body temperature to produce fertile sperm.

MALE REPRODUCTIVE SYSTEM

The ① **testes** are two oval glands and their functions are to produce sperm and the hormone testosterone. Sperm look rather like tadpoles and are produced continually from puberty until about 70 years of age. The ② **penis** contains the ③ **urethra**, which acts a passageway for both semen and urine.

Sperm pass along a coiled tube called the **epididymis**, which becomes wider to form the ④ **vas deferens**. The vas deferens is about 45 cm long and passes from the testes to the urethra. It acts as a passageway for sperm and has muscular walls to help to move sperm along. Each vas deferens passes through a sac-like gland called a **seminal vesicle** which releases fluid that makes up a substantial amount of semen. The **spermatic cord** supports the testes and contains the vas deferens, nerves and blood vessels.

The ⑤ **prostate gland** is about the size of a chestnut and lies under the bladder and surrounding the beginning of the urethra. It secretes a thin, milky fluid which is important for the normal functioning of the sperm cell and makes up about 25 per cent of the semen.

Note

A **gamete** is a sperm or ovum.

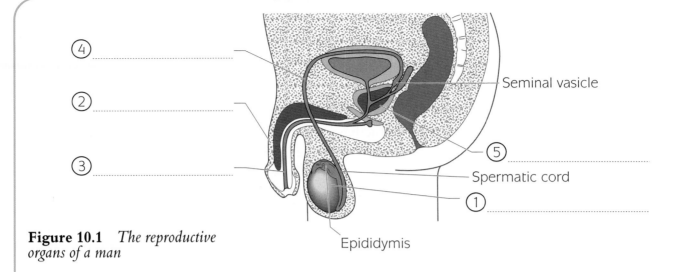

Figure 10.1 *The reproductive organs of a man*

Label the diagram in Figure 10.1 matching the numbers to the numbered terms in the text on page 169. Use this key to colour the diagram:

Red – teste

Orange – prostate gland

Yellow – urethra and vas deferens

Pink – penis.

FEMALE REPRODUCTIVE SYSTEM

The female reproductive system contains two ① **ovaries**, which are about 3 cm long. These glands are found either side of the uterus. Their function is to release the hormones oestrogen and progesterone and to produce ② **ova** (eggs).

When an ovum (egg) is released it enters the ③ **Fallopian tube**. The Fallopian tubes act as a passageway for sperm to reach the ovum and it is here that the ovum becomes fertilised.

The ovum enters the ④ **uterus** (womb) along the Fallopian tube. The pear-shaped uterus is located in the centre of the pelvic cavity, the bladder being in front and the rectum behind. The uterus connects with the vagina.

The ⑤ **cervix** (neck of the uterus) is a short and narrow passageway found at the bottom end of the uterus. It dilates during childbirth and the amount of dilation can be measured to decide how soon the baby will be born.

Note

If the ovum has been fertilised, a process known as **conception**, it attaches itself to the lining of the uterus. The fertilised ovum is now called a **zygote** and grows to become a baby. The gestation period is around 40 weeks.

Note

The **vulva** is the term used to describe the external female genitalia.

Fact!

Childbirth includes labour and delivery, and is also known as **parturition**.

The cervix opens into the ⑥ **vagina**, which serves as a passageway for childbirth and for menstrual flow.

The **perineum** is an area found between the opening of the vagina and the anus; muscles of the pelvic floor are attached to it.

Task 10.2

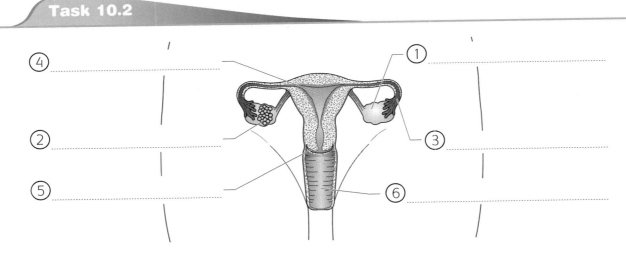

Figure 10.2 *The reproductive organs of a woman*

Label the diagram in Figure 10.2 matching the numbers to the numbered terms in the text above and on page 170. Use yellow to colour the ovaries and ova, and brown for the Fallopian tubes, uterus and cervix.

Fact!

The eggs carry the X chromosome but sperm may carry either an X or Y chromosome. If the sperm is carrying an X chromosome, the baby will be a girl. If it is carrying a Y chromosome, it will be a boy.

Fact!

The cervix dilates during childbirth and the amount of dilation can be measured to decide how soon the baby will be born.

Conditions associated with the female reproductive system

Polycystic ovarian syndrome

Ovarian cysts are usually harmless but can become large and painful and have to be removed. Larger cysts are often the result of hormonal imbalance and may cause the menstrual cycle to become irregular. In many cases it is due to high levels of male hormones, which can lead to excess hair growth.

Ectopic pregnancy

An ectopic pregnancy is one that occurs outside the uterus. The commonest place for this to occur is in the Fallopian tube. It is a very dangerous condition and can lead to internal bleeding.

The menstrual cycle

The pituitary gland, hypothalamus and ovaries play a part in controlling female reproduction. A typical menstrual cycle is about 28 days long. **Menstruation** (bleeding) lasts for about five days and is due to the thickened **endometrium** (lining of the uterus) breaking away. Oestrogens stimulate the growth of the endometrium and of follicles that encase the eggs (when fully grown they are known as **Graafian follicles**). An ovum (plural: ova) is produced and the uterus is prepared for pregnancy.

The release of an egg (**ovulation**) typically occurs around 14 days into the cycle. After ovulation, a structure called the **corpus luteum** forms from the ruptured follicle that had released the egg. It releases progesterone and oestrogen which stimulate continued thickening of the endometrium in preparation for possible pregnancy. If pregnancy does not occur, the corpus luteum begins to deteriorate causing progesterone and oestrogen levels to fall. Menstruation will begin once again.

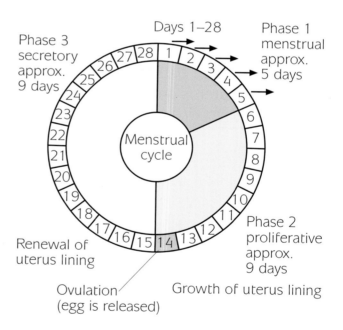

Figure 10.3 *The menstrual cycle*

Conditions associated with the menstrual cycle

Amenorrhoea
This is a condition in which menstruation stops, usually due to a hormonal imbalance. It can be due to obesity or extreme weight loss, such as someone suffering from anorexia nervosa.

Dysmenorrhoea
This is the term used to describe painful periods.

Premenstrual syndrome
Premenstrual syndrome (PMS) usually occurs one week before a period is due. Symptoms include irritability, fatigue, tearfulness and changes of mood. There may also be cramps, backache, bloating, fluid retention, and swollen and tender breasts. Women affected by PMS have a deficiency in serotonin (the body's own mood-uplifting chemical) during the premenstrual phase so are often prescribed antidepressants, which stimulate the release of these hormones.

THE BREAST

The function of the breasts is to produce milk (**lactation**) after childbirth. They lie over the pectoralis major and serratus anterior muscles and have a vast network of blood and lymphatic vessels. The breasts consist of glandular tissue, fibrous tissue and fatty (adipose) tissue.

Task 10.3

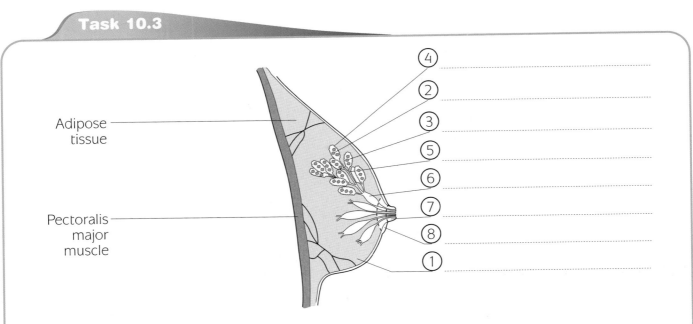

Figure 10.4   *The breast and its structures*

Label the diagram in Figure 10.4 matching the numbers to the numbered terms in the following text. Colour the diagram using yellow for the lobes, lobules, alveoli, milk ducts and lactiferous sinuses, and red for the Cooper's ligaments, areola and nipple.

Fact!

Cooper's ligaments become slack with age or with prolonged strain, such as long-term jogging, and can become irreversibly stretched, causing the breasts to sag.

① **Cooper's ligaments** are made up of strands of connective tissue and help to support the breasts. The ligaments become slack with age or with prolonged strain, such as long-term jogging, and can become irreversibly stretched, causing the breasts to sag.

A breast consists of about 20 ② **lobes** and each lobe contains several ③ **lobules**. The lobules contain milk-secreting glands called ④ **alveoli**. The ⑤ **milk ducts** carry the milk from the lobes and expand to form ⑥ **lactiferous sinuses**.

The lactiferous sinuses are found near the ⑦ **nipple** and act as storage for milk. The milk then passes into ducts to be released by the nipple. A pigmented area called the ⑧ **areola** (ah-ree-o-lah) surrounds the nipple and appears rough because of the presence of sebaceous glands which lubricate the nipple during suckling.

Blood supply and lymphatic drainage of the breasts

The subclavian and axillary arteries supply blood to the breast. The lymphatic drainage of the breast is extensive and leads mostly into the axillary lymph vessels and nodes under the armpits (Figure 10.5).

Note

If breast cancer develops, this extensive lymph drainage allows the cancer to spread elsewhere in the body.

Blood supply to breast

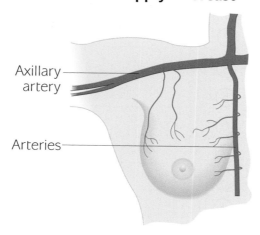

Axillary artery

Arteries

Lymph drainage of breast

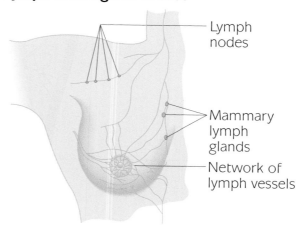

Lymph nodes

Mammary lymph glands

Network of lymph vessels

Figure 10.5 *Blood supply and lymph drainage of the breast*

Puberty

In the female, the breasts are quite flat until puberty. During puberty, breast development is stimulated by the hormones oestrogen and progesterone. **Oestrogen** stimulates the growth of the ducts and **progesterone** stimulates the growth of the alveoli.

These hormones cause additional adipose tissue to be laid down and the nipple and areola to increase in size.

During menstruation, the hormone **progesterone** causes increased blood flow to the breasts. This results in the retention of fluid in the breasts, causing them to increase in size. This usually happens shortly before a period and can cause discomfort for some women.

Pregnancy

After the baby is born, the hormone **prolactin** from the anterior pituitary stimulates the breasts to produce milk. The hormone **oxytocin** from the posterior pituitary affects the muscles in the walls of the alveoli, forcing milk to flow from the breasts. Milk is released in response to the suckling of a baby on the mother's nipple. Nerve impulses pass to the hypothalamus in the brain. The hypothalamus signals the anterior pituitary to release prolactin and the posterior pituitary to release oxytocin.

Menopause

During the menopause the production of oestrogen decreases and after the menopause oestrogen production stops altogether for most women. The lack of oestrogen causes changes to the body such as shrinkage of the breasts due to loss of glandular and adipose tissue. The supporting ligaments lose their strength and so the breasts sag.

The urinary system

11

The urinary system filters the blood and produces urine to ensure that the body gets rid of unwanted substances that could be harmful. It consists of two ① **kidneys**, two ② **ureters**, the ③ **bladder** and the ④ **urethra**.

Task 11.1

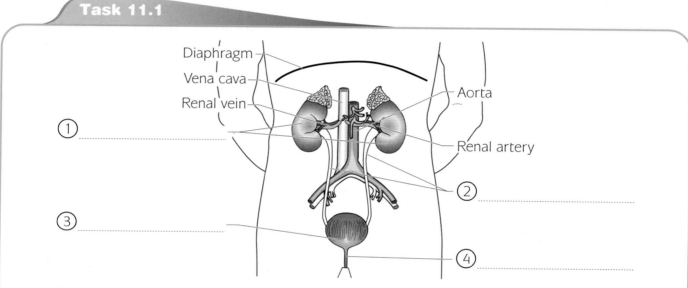

Figure 11.1 *The urinary system*

Label the diagram in Figure 11.1 matching the numbers to the numbered terms in the text above. Use this key to colour the diagram:

Brown – kidneys and ureters
Yellow – bladder and urethra

Red – arteries
Blue – veins.

THE KIDNEYS

The kidneys are two bean-shaped organs. Each would almost cover the area of a small hand and is about 2 cm thick. They are positioned in the lower back, mostly protected by the ribs, and are surrounded by a thick layer of fat.

The kidney is divided into the outer **cortex** and the inner **medulla**. The medulla contains about 14 triangular-shaped **pyramids**. The tip of each pyramid contains a cup-shaped **calyx**, which opens into the **renal pelvis**.

The word 'renal' means 'belonging to the kidney'. The renal pelvis is an open space that connects the medulla to the ureter. The **renal artery** and **renal vein** carry blood to and from the kidneys (Figure 11.2).

Fact!

The right kidney is slightly lower than the left because of the large space occupied by the liver.

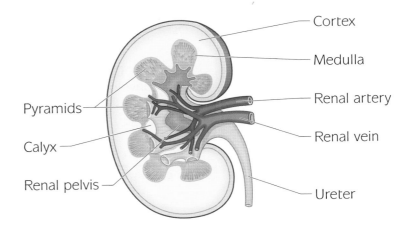

Figure 11.2 *View inside a kidney*

Functions of the kidney

The functions of the kidneys are to:

- filter the blood; in other words, to clean it and get rid of any unwanted substances (waste). Many of these substances are toxic and would result in death if they were allowed to accumulate in the body
- control the balance of water, salt and potassium in the body
- release hormones; one of these helps to produce vitamin D and the other stimulates the production of red blood cells
- help control blood pressure by controlling the blood volume in the body and by releasing an enzyme called **renin**
- control blood pH (acid/alkaline level). The normal pH of the blood is around 7.4. All the enzymes in the body can only work if the normal pH is maintained.

Fact!

In the average day, a kidney filters 1,300 litres of blood.

Filtering the blood

A kidney contains about a million filtration units called **nephrons** (nef'-rons) in which urine is formed. There are three parts to a nephron:

- the **proximal convoluted tubule**
- the loop of **Henle**
- the **distal convoluted tubule**.

Each nephron is joined to a **collecting duct**. The convoluted tubules of the nephron lie in the cortex, and the loops of Henle and collecting ducts lie in the medulla. The collecting ducts open into the renal pelvis (Figure 11.3).

Fact!

A kidney contains about a million filtration units called **nephrons** in which urine is formed.

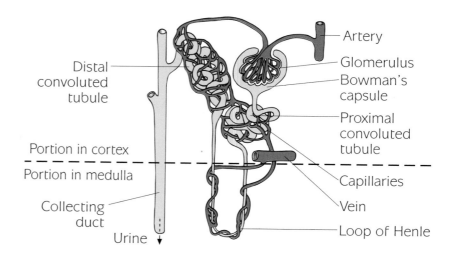

Figure 11.3 *Structure of a nephron*

Note

Blood cells and proteins are too big to pass through the capillary walls so remain within the bloodstream.

Ultrafiltration

Blood enters the nephron through bundles of capillaries called the **glomerulus** (glow-mer'-you-lus). The glomerulus is surrounded by the **Bowman's capsule**. The blood is brought at high pressure to the nephron, so water, amino acids, salt, glucose and waste products, such as urea, are squeezed through the walls of the blood vessels into the Bowman's capsule.

Reabsorption

The resulting fluid flows along the nephron and substances needed by the body, such as glucose, amino acids, salt and most of the water, are reabsorbed back into the bloodstream through nearby capillaries. The remaining water and waste products eventually reach the collecting duct of the nephron and become **urine**. The urine passes into the pelvis of the kidney. Waves of contraction in the pelvis walls force the urine into the ureter, which then passes it into the bladder.

Waste products

Unlike iron and certain vitamins, the liver cannot store excess proteins. The liver breaks down these extra proteins, which results in the formation of a waste product called **urea**. Urea is toxic to the body and is passed into the bloodstream to be filtered by the kidneys and excreted in the urine. The kidneys also excrete other waste products called **creatinine** and **uric acid**.

Control of fluid balance

Two-thirds of the body is made up of water, which is provided by the food and drink we consume. It is excreted from the body through urine, faeces, sweat and the breath. It is important for the body to balance the amount of water coming in with the amount of water leaving it.

The kidneys help to control this balance by removing water from the blood vessels that enter them and producing urine. They do this without affecting the other important substances in the blood.

The kidneys, under the influence of a hormone called **antidiuretic hormone** (see Chapter 8), control the amount of water excreted from the body. When extra water is needed by the body, for instance on a hot day when there is increased sweating and little water is drunk, the kidneys return (reabsorb) water into the bloodstream rather than releasing it as urine. This ensures that the balance of water in the body is maintained (see Chapter 8). When there is too much water in the body, the kidneys release it as urine.

Control of salt levels

Sodium (salt) is taken into the body through food and absorbed into the bloodstream. If there is too much sodium in the body, such as after eating a salty meal, the kidneys remove the excess from the blood. This restores sodium levels to normal. Eating too much salt tends to raise the blood pressure and results in an increase in urine output. The amount of sodium excreted by the body is controlled by the hormone **aldosterone** from the adrenal gland.

Control of potassium levels

Potassium is a mineral mostly found inside cells. It has many functions which include:

Fact!

Two-thirds of the body is made up of water, which is provided by the food and drink we consume.

Note

Drinking lots of water and producing little sweat results in pale and dilute urine. Drinking little water and excreting excess sweat produces less urine and that urine is more concentrated and darker in colour.

- maintaining proper acid/alkaline balance in the body
- helping with the passing of nerve impulses
- enabling muscle contraction to take place.

The hormone aldosterone also helps to control the levels of potassium in the body.

THE URETERS

Urine is formed in the kidneys and consists of 95 per cent water, 2 per cent mineral salts and 3 per cent waste products. It passes from the kidneys into two tubes called the **ureters**. The ureters are about 30 cm long and join on to the back of the bladder. The colour of the urine is produced by a bile pigment called bilirubin.

THE BLADDER

Urine is stored in a muscular sac called the bladder. When a sufficient amount of urine is collected in the bladder, the desire to urinate (**micturate**) will be produced. The bladder wall contracts and a sphincter muscle at the base of the bladder relaxes. Fortunately the release of urine can be controlled voluntarily by another sphincter muscle found at the bottom of the urethra. Small children do not have voluntary control over this particular sphincter muscle, hence the need for nappies.

THE URETHRA

The urethra is a narrow tube leading from the bladder to outside the body and is shorter in females than males. It acts as a passageway for urine and for sperm in males.

MASSAGE AND THE URINARY SYSTEM

The kidneys are mostly protected by the ribs and by muscles and are deeply embedded in fat. They are delicate organs so care has to be taken when massaging so as not to apply too much pressure.

Conditions associated with the urinary system

Kidney stones

Urine contains many salts and if little urine is being produced, like salt water left to evaporate, these salts can crystallise. More and more of the salts crystallise and form layers until a stone is made.

A small stone can enter the ureter and cause severe pain. It may pass naturally or surgery may be required to remove it.

Glomerulonephritis

A bacterial infection may lead to this condition in which the body's antibodies attack the glomeruli. There is inflammation of the walls of the glomeruli which causes the permeability of these walls to increase. Therefore, blood cells and protein, which usually stay within the capillaries, are able to pass into the urine. Symptoms include swelling of the tissues of the body (oedema), loss of appetite, vomiting and headache. The glomeruli may be permanently damaged, leading to kidney failure.

Cystitis

This is an infection of the bladder lining often caused by a bacterial infection. It is more common in women than men because of the shortness of the woman's urethra.

Crosswords

1 Cells

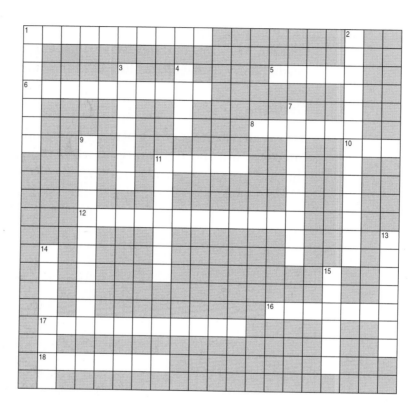

Across

1. The sum total of all the chemical reactions necessary to maintain life (10)
5. A by-product of cellular respiration (5)
6. Small organs (10)
8. Cells require this to burn up food (6)
10. Chromosomes consist of strings of ___ (3)
11. 'Body' responsible for sorting and packaging the proteins in the cell (5)
12. Powerhouses that help to produce energy for the cell (12)
16. Big groups of cells form these (7)
17. Chemical breakdown of foods by the cell is called cellular ___ (11)
18. Controls the cell's activities (7)

Down

1. Cell division (7)
2. A by-product of cellular respiration (6, 7)
3. Protein found in hair and nails (7)
4. One of the 100, 000 billion that make up the body (4)
7. Jelly-like liquid that contains nutrients for growth, division and repair of the cell (9)
9. These carry all the information needed to make an entire human being (11)
11. The fuel mostly used by the cell to produce energy (7)
13. Movement of water particles from high concentration of water to a low concentration through a partially permeable membrane (7)
14. Diffusion takes places through this, the cell ___ (8)
15. Tissue that contains many mitochondria (6)

2 Tissues

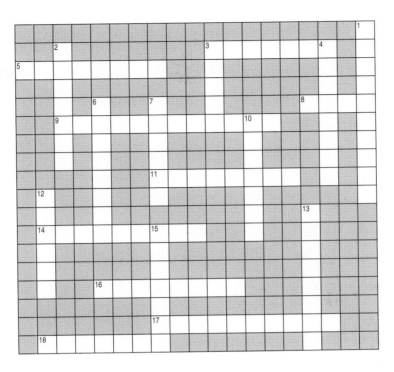

Across

3. Tissue found in muscle, bones, tendons and ligaments and made of collagen fibres (7)
5. Type of epithelium consisting of tall, column-shaped cells that lines the gallbladder and nearly all of the digestive tract (8)
8. Contains calcium phosphate to give this tissue rigidity (4)
9. Type of epithelium that lines the bladder and helps to prevent rupture of organs (12)
11. Tissue found in the lymph nodes and the spleen (8)
14. There are three types and fibro___ is one of them (9)
16. This type of epithelium consists of two or more layers (8)
17. This type of epithelium forms the top five layers of the skin (10)
18. A type of cartilage found at joints, where it reduces friction and shock (7)

Down

1. The function of this tissue is to protect, bind and support (10)
2. Type of tissue found where elasticity is needed, e.g. in the blood vessels (7)
3. Type of cartilage found where strength is required, e.g. in the discs between the backbones (5)
4. This type of membrane produces a thick fluid that lubricates the ends of bones (8)
6. Simple type of epithelium that is thin to allow rapid movement of substances through it (8)
7. Three types of tissue consisting of a single layer of cells (6)
10. This type of connective tissue is widely distributed throughout the body (7)
12. Type of membrane lubricated by a slimy, sticky fluid (6)
13. This type of tissue has the addition of fine, hair-like structures called cilia (8)
15. Fatty tissue found in most parts of the body (7)

3 Hair

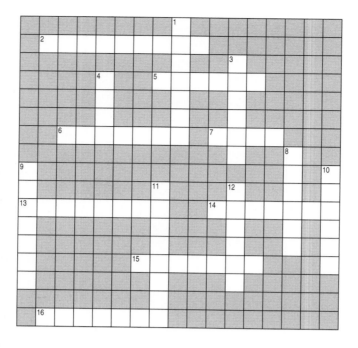

Across

2. Deep pits that extend into the dermis (9)
5. Layer of hair that contains pigment (6)
6. Hairs are made up of this (7)
7. Part of hair made up of lower and upper part (4)
13. Type of hair found on the head, underarms and pubic region (8)
14. Transitional stage of hair growth (7)
15. Determines the colour of hair (7)
16. Inner part of hair, not always present (7)

Down

1. Stage of hair growth in which the hair is resting (7)
3. Soft, downy hair found all over the body (6)
4. Consists of three layers (4)
8. Active growing stage of hair growth (6)
9. Outer part of hair (7)
10. Hair found on fetus (6)
11. Loss of hair (8)
12. Place where cells divide to produce hair (6)

4 Skeleton

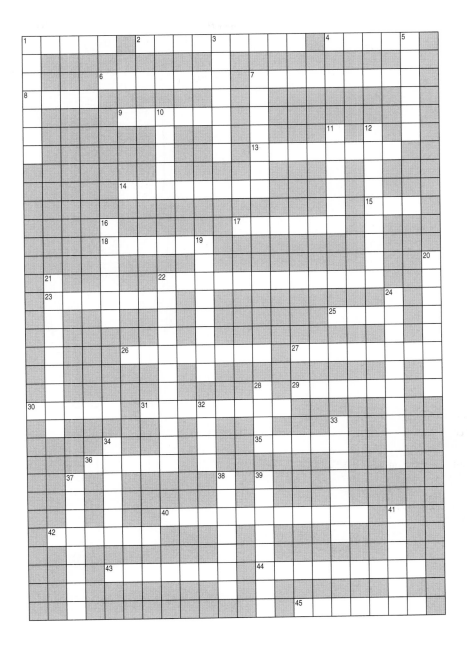

Refer to Figures 1 and 2 of the skeleton, the skull and the spine for the answers to the clues.

Across

1. See Figure 1 (5)
2. See Figure 1 (9)
4. See Figure 1 (5)
6. Hard, dense bone tissue that forms the outer layer of all bones (7)
7. Term to describe back of the body (9)
8. See Figure 1 (4)
9. Further away from the midline of the body (6)
13. See Figure 1 (8)
14. Term to describe the front of the body (8)
15. A function of the skeleton, produces this kind of blood cell (among others) (3)
17. The chest region (6)
18. See Figure 1 (6)
22. The formation of bone (12)
23. See Figure 1 (7)
25. See Figure 1 (4)
26. Closest to midline, in limbs it is the part nearest to the trunk (8)
27. See Figure 2 (8)
29. Towards the midline of the body (6)
30. See Figure 1 (5)
31. See Figure 1 (8)

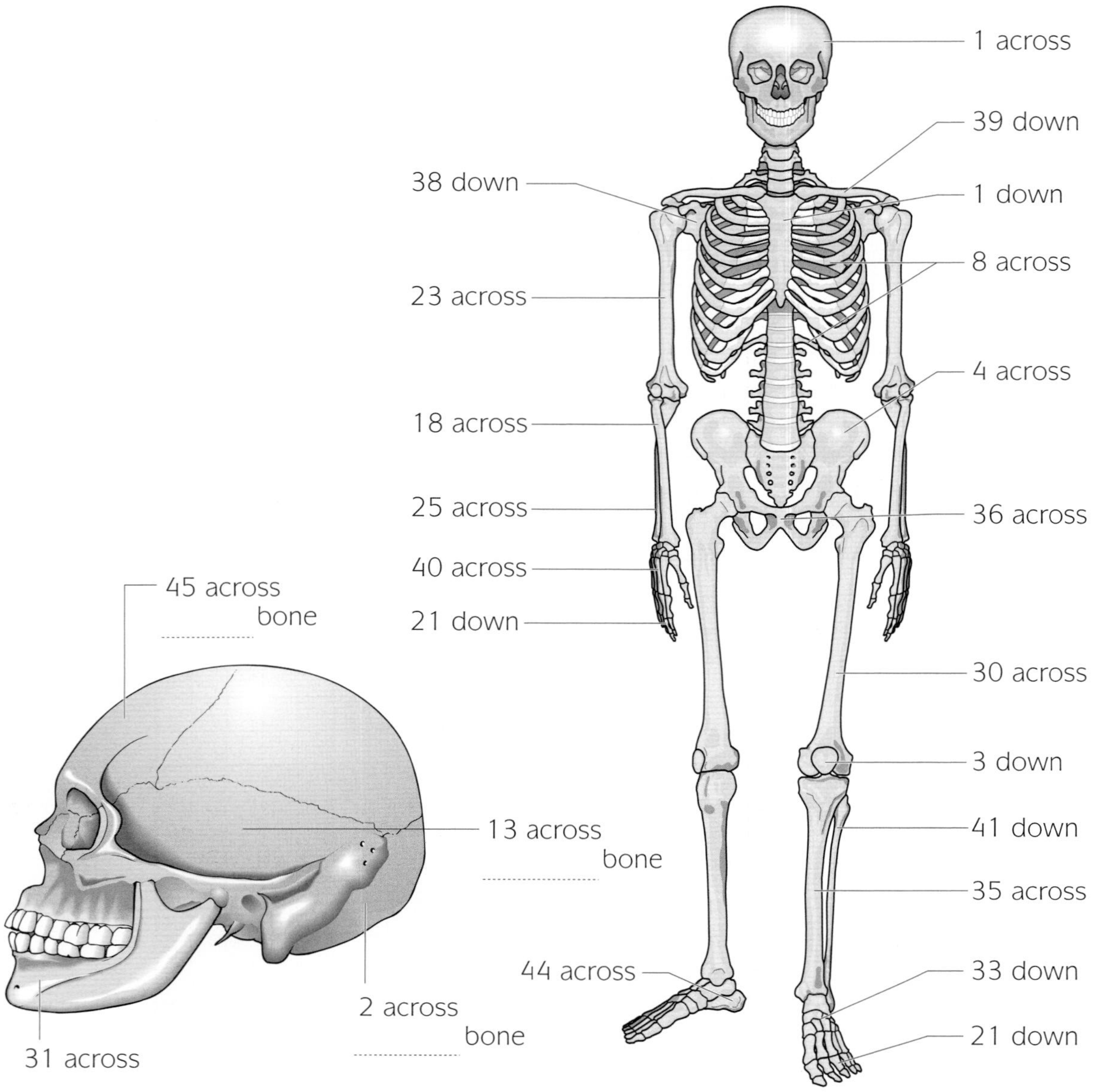
1 across
39 down
38 down
1 down
8 across
23 across
4 across
18 across
25 across
36 across
40 across
45 across
bone
21 down
30 across
3 down
13 across
bone
41 down
35 across
44 across
33 down
2 across
bone
21 down
31 across

Figure 1 *The skeleton*

Across (continued)

35. See Figure 1 (5)
36. See Figure 1 (5)
40. See Figure 1 (11)
42. See Figure 2 (6)
43. Towards the outer side, or away from the midline of the body (7)
44. See Figure 1 (9)
45. See Figure 1 (7)

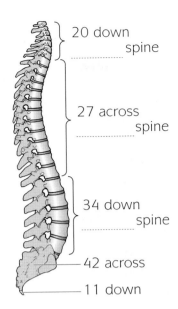

20 down _____ spine

27 across _____ spine

34 down _____ spine

42 across

11 down

Figure 2 *The spine*

Down

1. See Figure 1 (7)
3. See Figure 1 (7)
5. Found in cancellous bone and produces red blood cells (6)
7. On or towards the soles of the feet (7)
10. Type of bone found in wrist and ankles (5)
11. See Figure 2 (6)
12. A type of system found in compact bone (9)
16. Consist of medial longitudinal, lateral longitudinal and transverse (6)
19. Small rounded bones formed in tendon, found at the knee-cap (8)
20. See Figure 2 (8)
21. See Figure 1 (9)
22. Bone-building cells (11)
24. Bone tissue known as spongy bone (10)
28. Type of bone, such as the skull, which helps to protect organs (4)
32. Away from the surface of the body (4)
33. See Figure 1 (7)
34. See Figure 2 (6)
37. Attaches bone to bone to help prevent dislocation (8)
38. See Figure 1 (7)
39. See Figure 1 (8)
41. See Figure 1 (6)

5 Muscles

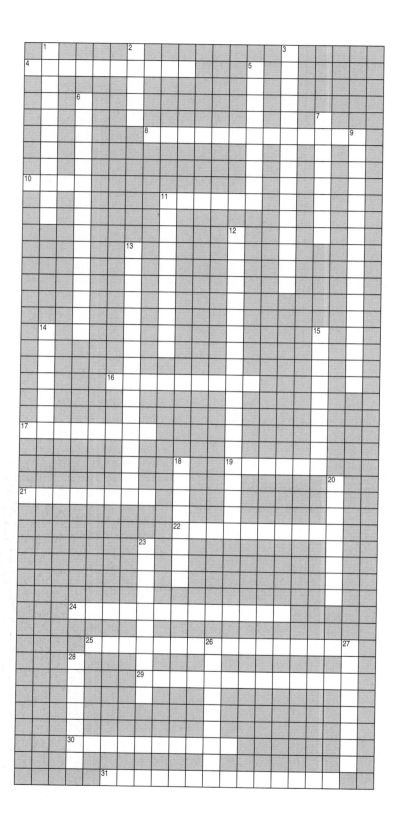

Refer to Figures 3, 4 and 5 for the answers to all the clues.

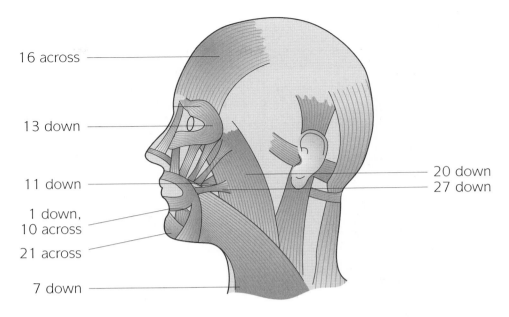

Figure 3 *Muscles of the face*

16 across
13 down
11 down
1 down, 10 across
21 across
7 down
20 down
27 down

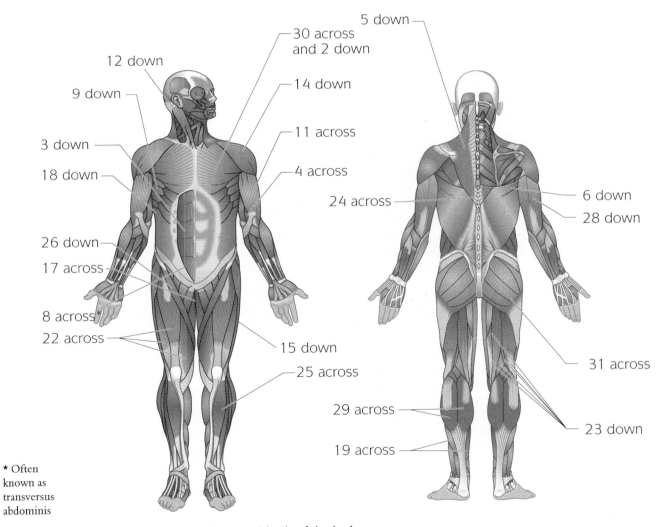

5 down
30 across and 2 down
14 down
11 across
4 across
12 down
9 down
3 down
18 down
24 across
6 down
28 down
26 down
17 across
8 across*
22 across
15 down
25 across
31 across
29 across
23 down
19 across

★ Often known as transversus abdominis

Figures 4 and 5 *Muscles of the front and back of the body*

6 Blood circulation

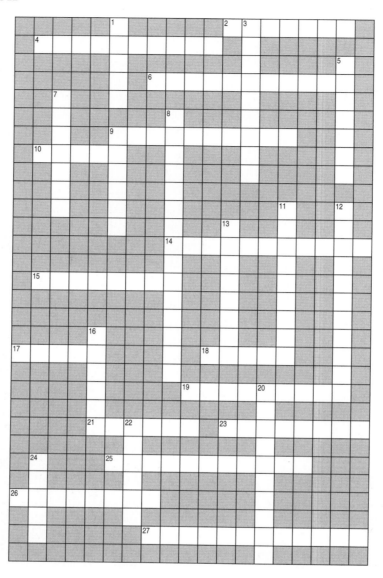

Across

2. Pulse can be felt in this artery in the neck (7)
4. Blood rich in oxygen (10)
6. A condition is which blood pressure is continually low (11)
9. Lower two chambers of the heart (10)
10. Upper two chambers of the heart (5)
14. Vessels that unite arterioles and venules (11)
15. Smoking, obesity and lack of exercise can lead to high blood ___ (8)
17. These blood cells protect us from disease (5)

18. Blood vessels that carry deoxygenated blood towards the heart (5)
19. Type of cancer caused by the overproduction of leucocytes (9)
21. Wall that separates left side of heart from the right side (6)
23. These mostly carry oxygenated blood away from the heart (8)
25. Red blood cells contain this pigment (11)
26. Reddening of the skin (8)
27. Condition in which blood pressure is consistently high (12)

1. The function of this muscle is to pump blood around the body (5)
3. This hormone causes the heart rate to speed up (9)
5. Lack of iron in the diet can lead to this condition (7)
7. Contraction of the heart (7)
8. Furring up of the arteries (15)
9. These help to prevent the backflow of blood (6)
11. The function of these blood cells is to clot the blood (9)

12. A blood disorder in which blood does not clot normally (11)
13. Relaxation of the heart (8)
16. Blood in the veins is called the ___ flow (6)
20. Lymphocytes produce these to destroy harmful bacteria (10)
22. The liquid part of the blood (6)
24. The largest artery of the body (5)

7 Lymph

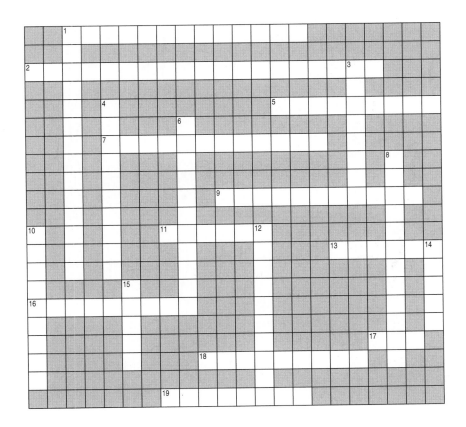

Refer to Figure 6 for the answers to the clues.

Across

1. See Figure 6 (13)
2. See Figure 6 (11, 8)
5. See Figure 6 (9)
7. See Figure 6 (8, 4)
9. Specialised white blood cells (11)

11. Lymphatic vessels contain these to prevent the backflow of lymph (6)
13. Organ made from lymphatic tissue (6)
16. Specialised white blood cells (9)
17. Nutrient that is passed from the small intestine into the lymphatic system (3)
18. See Figure 6 (9)
19. See Figure 6 (8)

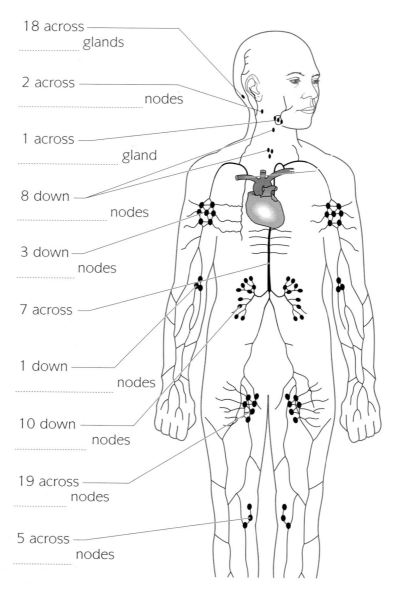

18 across _____ glands

2 across _____ nodes

1 across _____ gland

8 down _____ nodes

3 down _____ nodes

7 across _____

1 down _____ nodes

10 down _____ nodes

19 across _____ nodes

5 across _____ nodes

Figure 6 *Lymph glands of the body*

Down

1. See Figure 6 (14)
3. See Figure 6 (8)
4. Helps to stop the growth of bacteria and their harmful action (10)
6. Blind-ended tubes which tissue fluid passes into, lymphatic ___ (11)

8. See Figure 6 (4, 8)
10. See Figure 6 (9)
12. Lymph drains into these veins (10)
14. These filter harmful substances and inflame during infection (5)
15. Watery fluid that resembles plasma (5)

8 The respiratory system

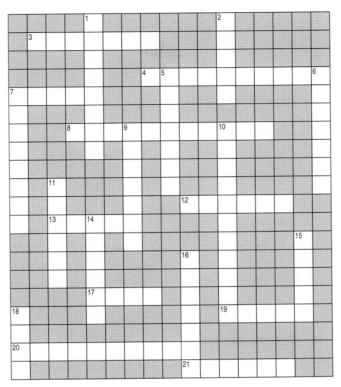

Across

3. These ensure an efficient gaseous exchange in the lungs (7)
4. Flap of cartilage which helps to prevent choking (10)
7. Hay___ – allergy causing runny nose and sneezing (5)
8. Breathing in (11)
12. Waste product produced by cells, ___ dioxide (6)
13. Tiny hair like structures (5)
17. Warms and moisten the air before it enters the pharynx (4)
19. Two of these are found in the thorax (5)
20. One of the tubes that branch off from the bronchi (10)
21. Condition that causes the muscles of the bronchi to constrict (6)

Down

1. The lungs are enclosed by a pleural ___ (8)
2. Goblet ___ produce mucus (5)
5. The throat (7)
6. Air-filled spaces found behind the nose and eyes (7)
7. When the diaphragm contracts it ___ (8)
9. Cavity surrounding lungs that contains fluid (7)
10. These muscles contract to lift ribs up and out (11)
11. The sinuses are lined with this type of membrane (6)
14. Voice box (6)
15. Bronchi contain ___ of cartilage to keep the tubes open and rigid (5)
16. Windpipe (7)
18. Bones that assist with breathing (4)

9 The nervous system

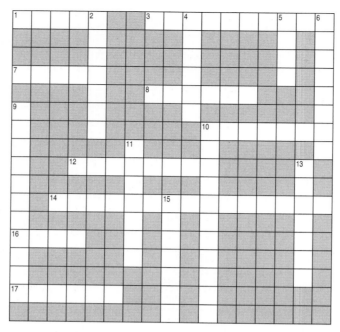

Across

1. The CNS is made up of the spinal cord and ___ (5)
3. Region of brain involved with balance and muscle co-ordination (10)
7. Nerves that conduct impulses from the CNS to a muscle or gland (5)
8. The fatty sheath around nerve fibres (6)
10. Small gap between two nerve cells (7)
12. Part of brain concerned with memory and learning (8)
14. Part of autonomic nervous system that prepares the body for rest (15)
16. The nerve fibre of a neurone (4)
17. Nerve fibres that extend from the brain through the vertebral column are called the ___ cord (6)

Down

2. Another word for a nerve cell (6)
4. A response that helps protect us from danger is called a ___ action (6)
5. Side of brain that mostly deals with scientific and numerical skills (4)
6. Membranes that enclose the CNS (8)
9. Maintenance of a constant internal environment (11)
10. Part of autonomic nervous system that prepares the body for action (11)
11. Nerves that conduct impulses from a sense organ to the CNS (7)
13. Nerves that supply muscles of the legs and feet (7)
15. Part of brain that regulates breathing and the heart beat, the ___ oblongata (7)

10 Hormones

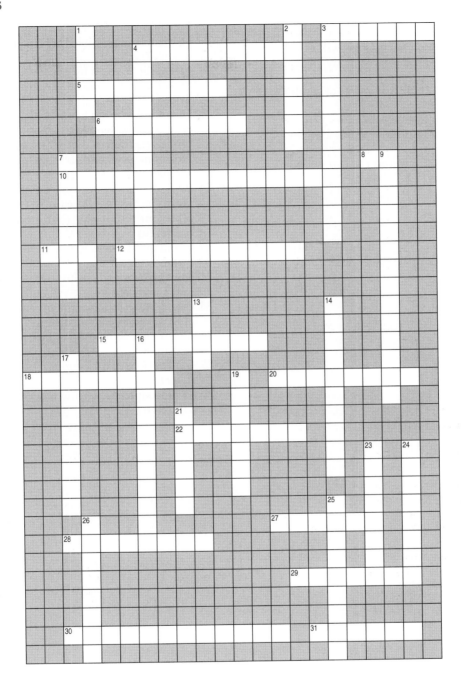

Across

3. Gland that releases hormone called melatonin (6)
4. Known as the 'fight or flight' hormone (9)
5. Hormone responsible for the release of milk from the breast during suckling (8)
6. Low levels of aldosterone and cortisol can lead to this disease (8)
8. Gonadotrophic hormone that stimulates ovaries to produce progesterone (2)
10. Symptoms of this condition include lose of weight, fast pulse and bulging eyes (15)
11. Gonadotrophic hormone that stimulates the ovaries to produce oestrogen (3)
12. A disease in which the bones thicken, causing enlargement of the hands, feet and face (10)
15. Master gland, controls most of the other glands (9)
18. Oversecretion of androgens can cause this condition in females (8)

20. Undersecretion of growth hormone can lead to this condition (8)
22. Glands that release hormones responsible for female sexual characteristics such as breast growth (7)
27. Increased sodium (salt) levels in the body can lead to this condition (6)
28. Disease caused by insufficient amounts of insulin in the body (8)
29. Two glands that sit on top of each kidney (7)
30. Overproduction of parathormone can lead to this condition (12)
31. Undersecretion of parathormone can cause this (6)

Down

1. Hormones are released directly into this (5)
2. Hormone responsible for bringing blood sugar levels down (7)
3. Hormone released by parathyroids (12)
4. Hormone that controls the amount of water released as urine (12)
7. Hormone released by thymus concerned with the production of lymphocytes (8)
9. Undersecretion of thyroxine causes this condition (14)
13. Hormone that controls the release of hormones from the adrenal cortex (4)
14. Body's own mood-lifting hormones (10)
16. Hormone produced by the testes (12)
17. Hormone responsible for the production of milk in the breasts (9)
19. Gland that releases hormone that controls the body's metabolism (7)
21. Mineral corticoids helps to keep a correct balance of this in the body (6)
23. Hormone that causes the liver and muscles to release glucose into the bloodstream (8)
24. Hormone that helps to reduce inflammation and feelings of pain (8)
25. Gynaecomastia is a condition affecting males and is due to increased levels of this hormone (9)
26. Overproduction of growth hormone can lead to this condition (8)

11 The digestive system

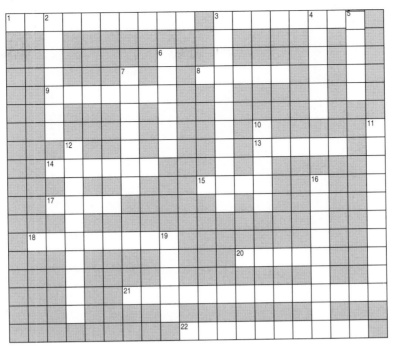

Across

1. Tube extending from the mouth to the stomach (10)
3. Gland that produces digestive enzymes and hormones (8)
8. Finger-like structures found on the inside of the small intestine (5)
9. Type of enzyme that digests starch (7)
13. The part of the small intestine after the jejunum (5)
14. Enzyme found in stomach, begins digestion of protein (6)
15. A greenish yellow liquid, helps with the digestion of fats (4)
17. A small bladder found attached to the liver (4)
18. The first part of the small intestine (8)
20. Absorbs water and mineral salts from the faeces (5)
21. A function of the liver (14)
22. If it is not ascending or descending it must be ___ (10)

Down

2. Large, curved bag that secretes gastric juices (7)
3. Wave-like contractions that help to move food through the alimentary canal (11)
4. Substance made from protein that speeds up chemical reactions (6)
5. The ___ intestine (5)
6. The indigestible matter remaining after digestion has taken place (6)
7. These juices contain hydrochloric acid and pepsin (7)
10. This organ produces bile and has many other functions (5)
11. The process whereby digested foods pass into the bloodstream (10)
12. All the chemical processes necessary for life, especially the cell's conversion of glucose into energy (10)
16. Ring of muscle found at both ends of the stomach (9)
19. The three pairs of salivary glands are found here (5)

12 The reproductive system

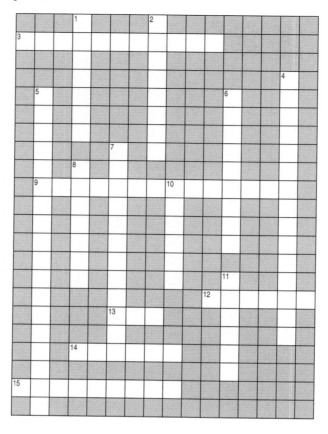

Across

3. Tube that acts as a passageway for sperm (3, 8)
9. Place where eggs are fertilised (9, 5)
12. Produce sperm and testosterone (6)
13. Ovaries produce these (3)
14. Fertilised egg attaches itself to the lining of this (6)
15. Lack of this hormone causes shrinkage of the breasts at menopause (9)

Down

1. Type of tissue found in breasts (7)
2. Gland that produces fluid that makes up part of the semen (8)
4. Helps to give support to the breasts (7, 8)
5. Acts as storage area for milk (11, 7)
6. Carries milk from lobes (4, 5)
7. Hormone involved with breast development at puberty (12)
8. Milk-secreting glands (7)
10. Pigmented area surrounding the nipple (6)
11. Narrow passage found at base of uterus (6)

13 The urinary system

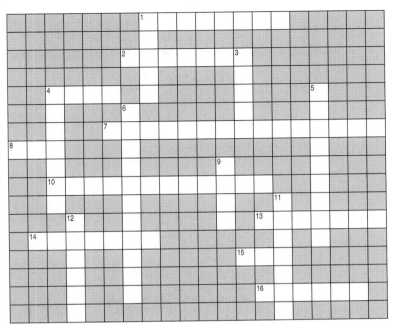

Across

1. Infection of the bladder lining, which can be caused by bacterial infection (8)
2. Muscular sac that acts as reservoir for urine (7)
4. Waste product, the result of protein breakdown (4)
7. Process whereby substances are squeezed from capillaries into Bowman's capsule (15)
8. Kidneys are deeply embedded in this (3)
10. Process whereby useful substances are passed back into the bloodstream from the nephron (12)
13. The inner part of the kidney (7)
14. Two tubes that urine is propelled through (7)
15. Hormone that controls the amount of water excreted from the body (3)
16. The outer part of the kidney (6)

Down

1. Found at the tip of each pyramid (5)
3. Artery and vein that carry blood to and from the kidney (5)
4. Acts as a passageway for urine and for sperm in males (7)
5. The kidney helps to control balance of this mineral in the body (9)
6. This hormone controls salt levels in the body (11)
9. Kidneys are partly protected by these bones (4)
11. A filtration unit in the kidney (7)
12. Cavity that connects the medulla to the ureter (6)

Index

Page references in *italics* indicate illustrations and those in **bold** indicate tables.

parathormone 148
parathyroid glands 142, *143*, 148
parietal bone 51, *52*
Parkinson's disease 141
paronychia 43
patella *56*, 57
pectoralis major *85*, **86**
pelvic girdle 55, *56*
penis 169, *170*
pepsin 160, 161
peptic ulcers 164
perineum 171, *171*
peripheral nervous system 132–8, *133–7*
peristalsis 159
Peyer's patches 113
phagocytes 92
phalanges 54, *55*, 57, *58*, 59
pharynx *115*, 116, *158*, 159
pH balance 7
phlebitis 103
pigmentation 15, 32–3
pineal gland 146
pinna *135*
pituitary gland 142–6, *143*, *144*, 146, 172, 175
pivot joint 62, *62*
platelets *92*, 93
platysma *74*, **75**
pleura 117, 122
plexuses of nerves 136, *136*
pneumonia 122
polycystic ovary syndrome 171
pons variolii *128*, 129
popliteal lymph nodes *110*, 111
posterior pituitary *143*, *144*, 145, 146, 175
posterior tibialis muscle *60*
posture 89–90
potassium 179–80
pregnancy 155, 171, 172, 175
premenstrual syndrome (PMS) 173
prickle cell layer of skin *13*, 14
prime mover muscle 76, *76*
progesterone 155, 172, 174, 175
prolactin 144, 175
pronation 63, *64*
pronator teres *81*, **82**
prostate gland 169, *170*
prothrombin 93
proximal convoluted tubule 178, *178*
psoas 79, **80**
psoriasis 36
pterygium 43
puberty 155, 174
pubis 55, *56*
pulmonary circulation 95, *96*, 100, *101*, *102*
pulse 106
pyramids of kidney 177, *177*

quadratus lumborum *79*, **80**
quadriceps femoris *87*, **88**

radius 54, *54*
Raynaud's disease 140
reabsorption 178
rectum *158*, 162
rectus abdominis *85*, **86**
red blood cells 91–2, *92*, 114
reflex action 137
renal vessels 100, *101*, *102*, 176, *176*, 177, *177*
rennin 177
repetitive strain injury 84
reproductive systems 169–75, *170–4*
respiration, cellular 3–4, *4*
respiratory system 115–22, *115*, *119*, *120*, 121–2
retina *134*
rhinitis 121
ribs 53, *54*, 120, *120*
right lymphatic duct *110*, 112, *113*
ringworm 30
risorius *74*, **75**
rosacea 35
rotation 63, *64*
rotator cuff 78

sacrum 57, 58, 135, *135*
saddle joint 62, *62*
salivary amylase 159
salt levels 179
sartorius *87*, **88**
scabies 31
scapula 53, *54*
scoliosis 90, *90*
seasonal affective disorder (SAD) 146
sebaceous glands *15*, 16, 21, 34–5, *38*
sebum 19
semi-circular canals *134*
seminal vesicle 169
sense organs 134, *134*
sensory nerves *15*, 17, *126*, 132
serous membrane 11, *11*, **11**
serratus anterior *85*, **86**
sesamoid bones 47, *48*, 55
sex corticoids 149–50
shingles 29
short bones 47, *48*
shoulder 53, *54*, 65, 77, 78, **78**
shunt vessels 107, *107*
sigmoid colon *158*, 162
sinuses *115*, 121
skeletal system 45–66
   bone types 47–8, *48*
   functions 45
   named bones 51–60, *52*, *54–60*
skin 13–44, *13*, *15*
   ageing 21–4, *22*
   cancer 36–7
   diseases and disorders 27–37, 40, 108
   functions 17, 19
   massage effects 20

tags 36
   types 24–6
small intestine *158*, 159–60, *160*
smell 122–4, *123*
smoking 23, 121
smooth muscle 67, *67*, 97
soleus *87*, **88**
spermatic cord 169
spinal cord 130–1
spinal nerves 134–6, *135*, 137
spleen 114
spongy bone *46*, 47
sprains 64
squamous layer of skin 36
sternocleidomastoid *74*, **75**
sternum 53, *54*, 120
steroids 23, 150–1
   oestrogen 49, 148, 150, 155–6, 172, 174, 175
   progesterone 155, 172, 174, 175
stomach *158*, 159
stratified epithelium 8, *13*, 14
styes 27
subclavian veins *110*
subcutaneous layer 13, *15*, 17
submandibular lymph nodes *110*, 111
subscapularis 77, **78**
sucrase 161
sugars 166, 168
superior vena cava 96, *96*, 99, 100, *102*
supination 63, *64*
supinator *83*, **84**
supratrochlear lymph nodes *110*, 111
sweat *15*, 16, 19, 179
sympathetic system 107, 138–9, **139**
synapses 126, *126*, 127
synovial joint 61, *61*, 62, *62*
synovial membrane 11, *11*, **11**
systemic circulation 95–104
systole 104, *105*

tachycardia 106
talus bone *58*, 59, *60*
tarsals 57
telogen hair growth 39, *40*
temperature 17, 19, 71, 130
temporal bone 51, *52*
temporalis *74*, **75**
tendons 50, *60*, 69
tennis elbow 50
tensor fasciae latae *87*, **88**
teres major/minor 77, **78**
terminal hair 39
testes 142, *143*, 156–7, 169, *170*
testosterone 49, 156–7
tetany 148
thalamus *128*, 129
thoracic duct *110*, 112
thorax 53, *54*, 57, 58
thrombocytes *92*, 93
thromboplastin 93